PRAISE FOR
Tris Dixon's *Damage: The Untold Story
of Brain Trauma in Boxing*

T0151728

"Anyone who loves boxing—even the sport's most die-hard supporters—must take a longer and more serious look at the issues that Tris Dixon writes about with such nuance and humanity in *Damage*. Having covered the NFL for two decades, I've seen increasing awareness of traumatic brain injuries. We need the same in boxing, for the fighters and their families, and there's no better argument for more studies, discussion, and awareness than this book, a volume equal parts heartbreaking and inspiring with respect to the need for change."
—Greg Bishop, *Sports Illustrated*

"[Aaron Pryor's] cautionary tale is told in Tris Dixon's fascinating new book, *Damage: The Untold Story of Brain Trauma in Boxing*. . . . Dixon's disturbing book ensures boxing no longer has any excuse."
—Dave Hannigan, *The Irish Times*

"Damage is an important book. . . . Tris Dixon writes well. . . . He's a meticulous researcher, which further elevates his work. . . . Dixon has made a major contribution to the health and safety of fighters. Now let's see who's paying attention."
—Thomas Hauser, Boxing Scene

"In his . . . groundbreaking *Damage*, Dixon documents the long-term effects that follow from eating thousands of brain-swirling blows."
—Gordon Marino, *The Daily Beast*

"I've often said while commentating for fights that a boxer's age should not be judged chronologically, but rather by the amount of punches he has taken. Tris Dixon's book *Damage* adds forensic proof to that statement, as he walks you and these fistic titans from the lights of the ring into the shadows of their dressing rooms. I highly recommend this book."
—Teddy Atlas, International Boxing Hall of Fame inductee, broadcaster, and author of *Atlas: From the Streets to the Ring: A Son's Struggle to Become a Man*

"A strong recommendation for *Damage*, by Tris Dixon. It is marvelously researched and beautifully written, and it's likely the most important book about boxing you're going to read."
—Steve Farhood, Showtime boxing analyst, and International Boxing Hall of Fame member

"In *Damage*, Tris Dixon has written an excellent book that is a must-read for everyone who is passionate about the sport of boxing. Dixon truly presents the viewpoints of all parties in a thorough fashion. Everyone should read this book—Commission staff, commentators, sports governing bodies, referees, doctors who work ringside, coaches, corner staff, and someone who works as a cutman but most importantly boxers and their families."
—Dr. Nitin Sethi, neurologist and member of the Association of Ringside Physicians and the Weill Cornell Concussion and Brain Injury Clinic

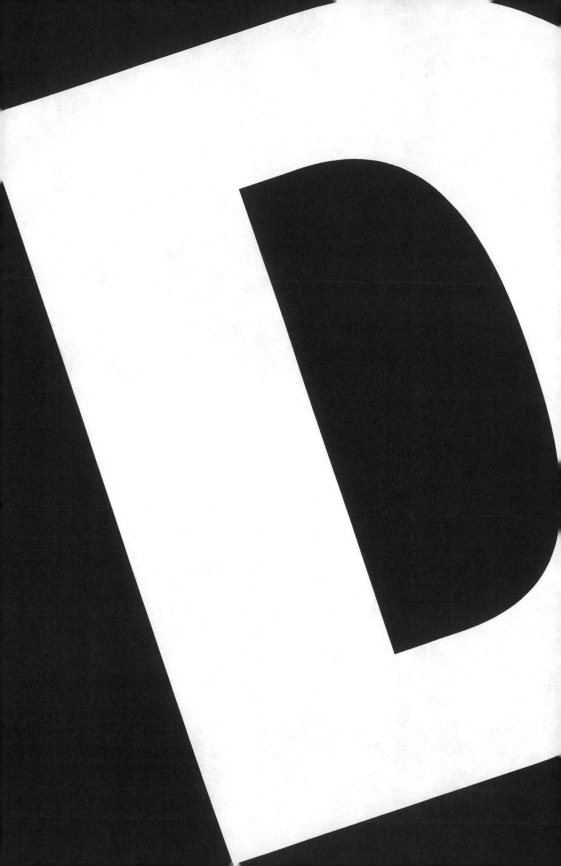

DA

MAGE

THE UNTOLD STORY
OF BRAIN TRAUMA
IN BOXING

TRIS
DIXON

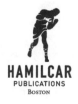

HAMILCAR
PUBLICATIONS
BOSTON

ISBN: 978-1-949590-53-1

Library of Congress Cataloging-in-Publication Data

Names: Dixon, Tris, author.
Title: Damage : the untold story of brain trauma in boxing / Tris Dixon.
Description: Includes bibliographical references. | Boston, MA: Hamilcar Publications, 2021.
Identifiers: LCCN: 2021934581 | ISBN: 9781949590531
Subjects: LCSH Boxing injuries. | Brain damage. | Brain—Wounds and injuries. | Brain—Concussion. | Sports injuries. | Sports—Safety measures. | BISAC SPORTS & RECREATION / Boxing | MEDICAL / Sports Medicine | MEDICAL / Neuroscience
Classification: LCC RC1220.B6 .D59 2021 | DDC 616.85/884—dc23

Hamilcar Publications
An imprint of Hannibal Boxing Media
Ten Post Office Square, 8th Floor South
Boston, MA 02109
www.hamilcarpubs.com

On the cover: Rocky Graziano punches Tony Janiro during their fight at Madison Square Garden on March 31, 1950.

For the fighters

CONTENTS

PROLOGUE . . . xiii

1 Punch-Drunk
ORIGINS OF A SPORTING EPIDEMIC . . . 1

2 Dementia Pugilistica
A DISEASE THAT DOESN'T DISCRIMINATE . . . 17

3 A Slick Medical Cliché
DENIERS AND DOUBTERS OF CTE . . . 33

4 The Collector
UNTOLD STORIES FROM THE BRAIN . . . 53

5 Poster Boys
A LABEL NOBODY WANTS . . . 65

6 Rusting Gold
BAD MEMORIES FROM A MAGNIFICENT ERA . . . 87

7 Concussion
THE NFL DENIED A CRISIS BOXING IGNORES . . . 99

8 The Study
A QUEST FOR ANSWERS . . . 127

9 Contradiction
A NEUROLOGIST AT RINGSIDE . . . 137

10 Chaos
BOXING'S ENDLESS PROBLEM . . . 147

11 Dilemma
A DAMAGED FIGHTER WONDERS WHETHER
HE SHOULD TRAIN BOXERS . . . 157

12 Buried Alive
"BOXING IS AMERICAN FOOTBALL HEAD INJURIES ON
STEROIDS" . . . 165

13 Labeled
"CTE SOUNDS A LOT BETTER THAN PUNCH-DRUNK" . . . 173

14 A Warrior's Brain
THE COST OF A PRICELESS LEGACY . . . 181

15 Trapped
FROM THE LIMELIGHT TO THE PSYCH WARD . . . 189

16 Risk Takers
DO FIGHTERS RECOGNIZE WHAT'S AT STAKE? . . . 199

17 Safety Nets
HELP AFTER THE FINAL BELL . . . 217

18 Tequila for Breakfast
SPARRING, QUITTING, RETIREMENT, DEPRESSION . . . 227

Epilogue
LOST . . . 235

Afterword
NOTHING FUCKS YOU HARDER THAN TIME . . . 251

REFERENCES 263
NOTES . . . 273
ACKNOWLEDGMENTS . . . 275

PROLOGUE

"I remember the shot. It was the opposite hand because I was facing him and I could see his glove coming over. And I'm walking over to him as if to say, 'Yeah, I'm going to get there before you.' And it wasn't like that. He got me. I didn't even flinch. Point blank."

Herol "Bomber" Graham holds an index finger to the right side of his face to show me where one of history's most spectacular punches detonated. "I was throwing an overhand right and he threw a bomb and it landed on here."

The punch, executed by the lethal middleweight Julian Jackson, saw Graham's body sway and then, with his lights turned out, plummet backward toward the canvas. Hard.

There were more bouts for Graham. More years of boxing, training camps, sparring, and fighting. There were victories and defeats, though nothing as epic as the thunderous Jackson blow that set in motion a chain of events that has resulted in Graham and I meeting in the psychiatric ward of a North London hospital.

It's a grim place. The summer sun shines, birds sing, and pigeons occasionally stop by a picnic table that has been bolted into the Astroturf, but even they don't stay for long. There is nothing to enjoy in the bleak surroundings. In the outdoor yard of the ward, empty shells of men who are trapped by the high walls for their safety and everyone else's roam during the afternoon. One murmurs to himself in the corner, facing the brickwork. Another, in his thirties and who could easily appear on the cover of

GQ, patrols the small area completing laps with a false confidence as if he is setting off on a mission. Another barks abruptly in an Eastern European accent. One resident sits alone in a trance. "He is the most unnerving," says one visitor. "He looks normal until he starts to talk." One comes up to shake my hand, then scuffles off before we can make contact. The patients take long, curious, tense looks at their visitors, but it's rude to stare back so they win every time.

It's an uneasy place to be, and I'm the least comfortable person here. There are plenty of staff members around, but the flat-screen TV on the wall is behind a protective cabinet for a reason. The residents who don't seem to be half asleep from medication have a twinkle of TNT in their eyes.

It doesn't seem like Graham belongs here. He's different, and not just because he challenged for a world title on three different occasions. He's like me. He greets me with a smile, asks about my trip, and escorts me outside to give us the best chance of being left alone.

He looks around at some of the forlorn faces. "I hope they don't go before me," he laughs, as if to say he must be in a bad way if they're released ahead of him. "That one," he adds, subtly raising his finger toward one lost soul, "I feel for him. He can't communicate with anyone. He doesn't know what he's doing."

I ask Graham what he's been up to, specifically what he did yesterday, and he racks his brain.

He doesn't know.

"That's how bad it is," he says, shaking his head. "Short-term memory loss. . . . I can remember things from years ago but yesterday. . . ."

He's trying to conjure images, clues, anything he can use to lever out information.

"Yesterday . . . I'm trying to think now. . . . It's from the McCallum fight. Not the McCallum fight. . . ."

He searches briefly for names. "The Jackson fight, especially. I mean, the shot he hit me with. I was out before I touched the floor. That was it. That was the beginning and end of it, if you know what I mean."

We sit side by side on a bench. He's wearing a tri-blend grey T-shirt with a chest pocket. He looks muscular. None of the other guys in the ward would want to go a couple of rounds with him, that's for certain. He knows I'm writing this book and is keen to talk about the damage he has sustained in boxing.

He arrives at the Jackson annihilation swiftly and unprompted.

"Everything changed from the one punch?" I ask him.

"Ah, you what?"

Graham, I find, has a habit of saying, "You what?" when he emphatically agrees with something.

"Big style. In a big way," he continues.

He asks if I can retrieve the fight on my phone, and within seconds we're watching the fateful fourth round. That seismic punch lands. He sighs loudly. The air leaves him.

"That's what we were worried about," screams Screensport commentator Dave Brenner.

"But I was still breathing anyway," Graham whispers, as though it was a moral victory.

"Did you feel it?"

"Ah, you what?"

He laughs uneasily. I assumed the punch could have been so hard and knocked him so stiff and so cold that it immediately had switched off any feelings.

"Come here, let me try it on you," he chuckles. "It hit the side of my face, I felt a numbness and I remember falling. I could feel myself going down." Then blackness.

The next thing Graham remembers is being in the hospital. "After that, I watched it on television and it was then I really felt it," he says. "Watching it, I felt it. I felt that punch."

"What happens now, seeing that and believing it caused you to be here today?" I ask him.

"It's like, shit. . . . If I did what I was supposed to have done for myself, which is run, run away. . . . But I went to him. And when you're going into a person the shot is twice as hard. Normally I'd back off and back off and back off."

How can Graham be sure that one strike caused years of depression and such an unstable disposition that he finds himself inside these four vacant walls, in a ward where staff attempt to protect him from an endless cycle of suicide attempts? Science would argue that it is the thousands of blows Graham took through his career—rather than just the one game changer—that is responsible.

"That fight in itself triggered it," he insists. "The one shot I got there was like all the shots I got in boxing combined, added up to a big one."

Whether it was the solitary blow or those accumulated in his fifty-four-fight career we cannot be sure. But he knows his being here is a result of the sport.

"It's . . . because of the trauma to my brain," he explains. "They said I got hit and all the blood vessels have exploded and all that type of stuff. It's a depression. Since then I've been in a depression. It's going to make me cry. . . ."

The tears suddenly stream down his cheeks. He hides his face in his hands and "Oh shit" comes from behind the guard.

He's hurt. He's embarrassed. He's alone. He indicates that he needs some time by raising his right hand. I place mine on his shoulder to comfort him.

"You see? That's how bad it is," he continues. "It's from boxing. Definitely. Definitely. I didn't get punched as much as a lot of them but it's enough in the sense it's hurt me and I've got brain damage. You do get punch-drunk. It does do that to you."

1

Punch-Drunk

ORIGINS OF A
SPORTING EPIDEMIC

"Leo Lomski, trying to finish it right here and now! Down he goes again! The champion is down!"

It was January 6, 1928, and Philadelphia's world light-heavyweight king Tommy Loughran was on the deck for a second time, seemingly about to lose his crown to Lomski. The challenger was one second from victory after Loughran, his brain scrambled by a thunderous right hand, rose at the count of nine once more.

Loughran was a boxing scientist with wonderful skills and a precise jab. He had managed to fend off Lomski's attacks, cutting Leo—who had broken his right hand during a fiery first-round assault—badly by the left eye before assuming control and winning on points over fifteen rounds.

It was a thriller: brutal, technical, bloody.

"This is one of the great comebacks in the history of the ring, with the champion down twice in the first round coming on strong," rejoiced the announcer.

The Ring, then in its infancy after first being published only six years earlier, voted the bout as Fight of the Year for 1928. Staged at New York's iconic Madison Square Garden, it had drama, seesaw action, and highlight-reel exchanges aplenty.

Fifteen miles away, however, in the less frenetic surroundings of the Newark Medical Center, an American pathologist named Harrison Martland was busy putting the finishing touches on an intensive study on boxing that would forever cast a dark shadow over the sport.

Martland had not been ringside for the Loughran–Lomski clash. Nor did he share any enthusiasm for the public excitement engendered by that epic struggle. Instead, he was analyzing the results of a number of boxing contests. He was not interested in points scored but in punches landed. More specifically, in the effects of the thousands of blows a professional boxer typically receives during his career. Through his studies, Martland hoped to evaluate the short- and long-term consequences of boxing on the physical and mental well-being of fighters.

Dr. Harrison Martland was born in 1883 during the reign of the first world heavyweight champion, John L. Sullivan. By the time Sullivan was no longer able to boast that he "could lick any sonofabitch in the house," Martland was a decade removed from earning a degree at West Maryland College. He added to that in 1905 with an M.D. degree from Columbia University.

In 1909, with Jack Johnson tearing through the heavyweight ranks, Martland became the first paid pathologist at Newark City Hospital. After a two-year term as president of the Essex County Medical Society, Martland became president of the Academy of Medicine in Northern New Jersey in 1922. He went on to win a battle in the state legislature in 1927 to change a system that had permitted a coroner's jury of laymen to render verdicts on sudden-death cases. Medical people needed to do it, Martland contended, and he was consequently appointed chief medical examiner. By 1928 he was named the first out-of-state president of the New York Pathological Association, and in 1933 he began a fifteen-year stint as professor of forensic medicine at New York University.

Martland earned countless awards and accolades throughout his career and, in 1943, he was honored with the Edward J. III Award by the Academy of Medicine. Following his death in 1954, the new city hospital in Newark was named the Harrison S. Martland Medical Center, which would become part of Rutgers University.

But back in 1928, after Loughran and Lomski delivered their feast of violence on a freezing night in New York City, Martland went to work. He wrote a medical paper entitled "Punch Drunk" and published it in the *Journal of the American Medical Association*. In doing so, he established the term "punch-drunk syndrome" in a medical context. Although the term had long been used by boxers, managers, and promoters, the phrase was largely unrecognized by the medical community. *Punch-drunk* used pejoratively described boxers who were losing their faculties in the form of slurred speech, awkward movement, memory loss, and other degenerative behavioral changes. Martland's exhaustive studies had the effect of connecting the dots. After 1928, *punch-drunk* would become a requisite term in the medical lexicon.

Martland's interest in boxing had begun when a promoter presented him with several subjects to examine as a routine part of his role as a medical examiner. He personally inspected five of the cases and received clinical details about the rest. "For some time fight fans and promoters have recognized a peculiar condition occurring among prizefighters which, in ring parlance, they speak of as 'punch drunk,'" began Martland in his paper. "Fighters in whom the early symptoms are well recognized are said by the fans to be 'cuckoo,' 'goofy,' 'cutting paper dolls,' or 'slug nutty.'"

In Germany, the condition was known as *weiche birne* (soft pear). In Italy it was *suanato come una compana* (ringing like a bell). Boxing commissions, too, were not unaware of the condition. In early 1914, in what might have been the first example of medical experts influencing boxing, the New York State Athletic Commission ruled to remove the boxing license of Bob Fitzsimmons, the former middleweight, heavyweight, and light-heavyweight world champion. Fitzsimmons, fifty-one years old and well beyond his best, chose to sue. The court, however, ruled against him, believing that if "Ruby Rob" was allowed to fight on he ran the risk of damaging himself and the sport.

Fourteen years later, Martland concluded that those most susceptible to punch-drunk syndrome were "poor boxers" prone to taking punishment as well as sparring partners—"second-rate fighters used for training purposes who may be knocked down several times a day."

Describing the physical signs of the syndrome, Martland wrote: "There may be only an occasional and very slight flopping of one foot or leg in walking, noticeable only at intervals; or a slight unsteadiness in gait or uncertainty in equilibrium. These may not seriously interfere with fighting. In fact, many who have only these early symptoms fight extremely well, and the slight staggering may be noticed only as they walk to their corners."

Martland acknowledged that movements became slower, that there were mood changes, that either one or both legs tended to drag while walking, the body swayed, there were tremors in hands and arms, and the "mental deterioration may set in necessitating commitment to an asylum." The pathologist then added: "The early symptoms of punch drunk are well-known to fight fans, and the gallery gods often shout 'Cuckoo!' at a fighter. I know of one fight that was stopped by the referee because he thought one of the fighters was intoxicated."

Martland suspected that around half of all participants could be at risk "if they keep at the game long enough."

"As far as I know this condition has practically not been described in medical literature. I am of the opinion that in punch drunk there is a very definite brain injury due to single or repeated blows on the head or jaw which cause multiple concussion hemorrhages in the deeper portions of the cerebrum," he wrote. Martland also noted the similarities with Parkinson's disease and said he felt it was his "duty to report this condition."

Coming as they did at a time when there was little or no official recognition of the long-term dangers inherent to boxing, Martland's conclusions were groundbreaking. What's more, he compiled his research in the absence of any existing medical records or statistical evidence with which he could substantiate his hypotheses. With great determination, Martland set about uncovering the dark truth behind the glamorous sport. After conducting numerous interviews with participants and those working behind the scenes in boxing, he concluded that punch-drunk syndrome was an open secret in the sport.

"We are placed in the position of accepting a series of objective symptoms described to us by laymen," Martland continued. "There is undoubted proof that for years fighters, fight promoters, and the sporting world have recognized and talked about this condition. . . . I have found that the opinion of shrewd laymen, many of whom are making a living by observing the physical fitness, actions, and characteristics of the professional fighter, is perhaps more substantial than the opinion of medical experts. A fight promoter whose ability to judge [that] the physical condition of fighters is unquestionable has given me the names of twenty-three fighters whom he considers punch drunk."

The boxers Martland alluded to were from all over the United States. Some had traveled to America from Europe, chasing fame and fortune. Four were now in asylums, undergoing treatment for unknown and undiagnosed illnesses. All of the five Martland examined from the pool of twenty-three exhibited symptoms that the pathologist believed were consistent with punch-drunk syndrome.

One subject, designated "CASE 2" by Martland, exhibited "advanced Parkinsonian syndrome due to punch drunk." Maybe because it was a medical paper, maybe because he did not have the family's consent, or maybe to protect the individual, CASE 2's identity was not published. But Martland left clues. He said the ex-fighter, whose initials were N. E., debuted in 1906, at the age of sixteen, and retired in 1913. He was a featherweight who had also boxed as a lightweight. He fought the likes of Jack Britton, Tommy Lang, Johnny Baker, Kid Burns, Charlie Griffin, Harry Stone, KO Brown, Tommy O'Toole and Teddy Maloney. CASE 2 had competed in good company; his best win was probably over Griffin. He had also lost a six-round decision to future Hall of Famer Britton.

Martland revealed CASE 2 had been knocked out twice, including once when he was twenty-two years old and "he was out for an hour." CASE 2 had suffered no previous illnesses, nor did he regularly drink alcohol. Despite this, the subject was frequently accused of being intoxicated because of the similarity of his symptoms with drunkenness. CASE 2 retired at age twenty-three because his left hand shook involuntarily and his legs were unsteady. Martland also indicated that there were problems with his speech because his tongue had a tremor.

Before his examination, CASE 2—"a well-nourished and healthy man"—had visited several clinics to find out what was happening to him. He had been assured that fighting didn't have anything to do with his condition.

People who knew boxing understood that CASE 2, or N. E., was turn-of-the-century Philadelphia slugger Nathan Ehrlich. Ehrlich was said to be a popular Jewish fighter but even today the city's preeminent boxing historians do not know much about him. Martland estimated—or had been told—that Ehrlich fought from 1906 to 1913; today's records show his career spanned from 1905 to 1911. The pathologist believed that Ehrlich had been knocked out twice, although some statistics contend it was three times. Martland believed Ehrlich was thirty-eight at the time of the study, although additional sources suggest that he would have been forty.

According to BoxRec, the boxing statistics website, Ehrlich fought six times in 1905, four times in 1908, twenty-seven times in 1909 (including seven bouts by the end of February), eleven times in 1910, and six times in 1911.

Years later, a relative writing online about "Uncle Nate" recalled how Ehrlich had one day witnessed "some boys beating up an old man." Ehrlich apparently intervened but was felled, hitting his head on the pavement, causing brain damage.

Such anecdotes have often served as a convenient means of clouding the very real damage that boxing can inflict on its participants. Indeed, fighters and their families have frequently been ridiculed by those unwilling to acknowledge the existence of punch-drunk syndrome.

In 1928, a benefit night in the form of a boxing event was held for Ehrlich in Philadelphia, although the history books do not record the reason for the nine-fight charity show at the Broadway Arena. Given the level of opponent that Ehrlich had competed against, it's revealing that little is known about the boxer. For Ehrlich was not just a fighter—he was much more than that. Although it wasn't recognized at the time, Ehrlich's importance to boxing cannot be underestimated: Nathan Ehrlich was the first recorded boxer medically diagnosed with punch-drunk syndrome. This gives him the unwelcome distinction of being boxing's bona fide patient zero. Had Ehrlich's plight not come to the attention of Martland, it's possible that hundreds of thousands of boxers may have continued to suffer in silence, ignored by medical authorities and subjected to derision and scorn.

Nathan Ehrlich died on January 5, 1957, just three years after Martland, but together they shared a unique history. Martland's "Punch Drunk" paper concluded that an autopsy conducted on most boxers was likely to reveal "multiple punctate hemorrhages in the deeper structures of the brain."

As the evidence of punch-drunk syndrome continued to mount, Martland urged medical authorities to address the problem. "The condition of punch drunk has been described," he emphatically concluded. "While most of the evidence supporting the existence of this condition is based at this time on the observations of fight fans, promoters, and sporting writers, the fact that nearly one-half of the fighters who have stayed in the game long enough develop this condition, either in a mild form or a severe and progressive form which often necessitates commitment to an asylum, warrants this report. The condition can no longer be ignored by the medical profession or the public. It is the duty of our profession to establish the existence or nonexistence of punch drunk by preparing accurate statistical data as to its incidence, careful neurologic examinations of fighters thought to be punch drunk, and careful histologic [tissue structure] examinations of the brains of those who have died with symptoms simulating the Parkinsonian syndrome. The late manifestations of punch drunk will be seen chiefly in the neurologic clinics and asylums, and such material will practically fall to the neuropathologist connected with such institutions."

In his seminal paper, Martland revealed—in tabular form—the initials of the twenty-three fighters who were in all probability suffering from punch-drunk syndrome. The pathologist provided more comprehensive research material on ten of the subjects in question. In total, fifteen boxers were said to be "punch drunk" while others had either "Parkinsonian syndrome" or were described as "drags left leg; bad shape" or "drags leg; talk slow." From the initials on display it was relatively easy to deduce that among the subjects were former lightweight champion Battling Nelson, heavyweight trial horse Joe Downey, Ukraine-born but Philadelphia-residing lightweight Joe Tiplitz, London-born and Philadelphia-based welterweight southpaw Bobby Barrett, Bronx lightweight Willie Jackson, the great lightweight Ad Wolgast, Dublin-born and New York–based Bartley Madden, and gutsy heavyweight Joe Grim.

"Punch Drunk" was a poignant and well-considered study that was difficult to ignore. In writing his paper Martland had used scientific research from New York neuropsychiatrists Michael Osnato and Vincent Giliberti, published the previous year, entitled "Postconcussion Neurosis—Traumatic Encephalitis" as well as C. B. Cassasa's paper "Multiple Traumatic Cerebral Hemorrhages." Osnato and Giliberti were the first scientists to propose that exposure to traumatic brain injuries, or TBIs, could lead to neurodegenerative changes. Their findings were presented at an annual meeting of the American Neurological Association in 1926.

In addition to this scientific research, Martland based his findings on the empirical testimony of boxing laymen as opposed to the theoretical speculations of self-proclaimed "experts" in the field of boxing-related injuries. The evidence of those who worked closely with fighters daily was powerful and persuasive. The science may not have existed entirely but if one cared to look in the right direction, the evidence was undeniable.

The problem was that fighters were winding up in asylums, hospitals, and sanatoriums and no one in the medical field really knew what was wrong with them. No one understood. For many fighters, the end result of this wholesale reluctance to address the issue of punch-drunk syndrome was that their symptoms were left to spiral out of control. The rest of the world chose to look the other way as countless victims of the sport were left to suffer in silence. They struggled with degenerating motor skills and cognitive functions. Many died tragically in middle age; others didn't even make it that far.

* * *

On the other side of the United States from Martland, in Verona, California, a former world lightweight champion was currently training for a comeback. Ad Wolgast, the "Michigan Wildcat," was one of the greats.

Before the First World War, Wolgast's wife had divorced him after he had squandered a $300,000 fortune. During the hearing, a Milwaukee court declared Wolgast "mentally incompetent." Wolgast was institutionalized but, amazingly, three years later, he was released from custody and allowed to fight Lee Morrisey in San Bernardino, California, in an exhibition.

According to reports, during the contest Wolgast "was hissed and booed and that ended his fistic career."

Two years later, he was flat broke and mentally wrecked. He was taken in by old fight manager Jack Doyle, repeatedly asking day after day, "When am I going to start sparring?"

"Tomorrow," Doyle, who had been given custodial responsibility of Wolgast, would assure him. Doyle instructed that no one in his gym could spar with his friend: "Let him continue to shadow box and punch the bag and do his road work, but no one is to hit him with a boxing glove."

Great fighters came to visit Wolgast, including Jim Jeffries, Tommy Ryan, Tom Sharkey, and Joe Rivers. They patted him on the back and told him he was the best, but he viewed the world through blank, bleak eyes that could only stare into the distance of a hazy rearview mirror.

Wolgast had lost his mind. He was labelled "insane" and institutionalized in Patton State Hospital, formerly Patton Asylum. Those who knew Wolgast's history believed that the issue was simple to explain: too many blows to the head.

After he was moved to Stockton State Hospital, Wolgast was prone to mood swings and rapid changes in behavior; at one point, two men ganged up on him and gave him the beating of his life. He was sixty-one and left blind. A few years later he was frail, gray, and in a wheelchair. Those who visited him estimated that only around 10 percent of any conversation made sense; the rest was errant rambling—about boxing, about his childhood in Michigan, about his fights.

"Out in California, there sits a pathetic figure in a State mental institution awaiting the call to his Heavenly Father," wrote Nat Fleischer, one of the great editors of *The Ring* magazine, who authored a four-part series on Wolgast through 1954. It made for grim reading. "Helpless, extremely ill, his mind all shattered, Ad Wolgast, the lightweight who made the headlines during the period between 1906 and 1916, the days when the world's greatest lightweights were performing, has again hit the extraordinary, but as a nationally famous personality whose days on this earth are numbered."

Fleischer, who in 1934 wrote that he knew of almost forty fighters who had been institutionalized for punch-drunkenness, reported how Wolgast's "memory was shattered," how he was occasionally dangerous and threatened to punch anyone who crossed him in the gym, and how he would "become wild." Wrote Fleischer: "He had reached a point where he was broken in everything but spirit, a victim of the ring game and all its trappings, doomed to semi-individualism for the remainder of his days."

Despite his condition, inside the California institution, Wolgast's training continued unabated—minus the roadwork, of course. But while the guards left him to it, other inmates did not. "They made life miserable as they termed him a 'punch drunk crazy fighter,'" continued Fleischer, who went to visit Wolgast one day for the series. The revered editor had been turned away because he was late but he did manage to speak with an attendant and the prognosis was stark.

"He's in a bad way," Fleischer was told. "He keeps working every day, shadow boxing and rope skipping without the aid of a rope, and his antics annoy those within range. He believes he will soon return to the ring to fight for the championship. Only recently a group of physicians, alienists, several newspapermen, and hospital attendants were watching regretfully while the graying little man feinted, hooked, side-stepped, swung vicious rights and lefts that landed in the air—all at an imaginary foe. He was giving a workout to prove that he would be ready for [Battling] Nelson in a few days. It was a pitiful sight. Those who watched were checking to see if he could be released, but he was too far gone. When he quit to rest, his head dropped into [his] arms as he sat on a bench, while down the corridor in the psychopathic ward one inmate kept shouting, 'you're goofy. The fellow's cuckoo. He's just crazy.'"

Unfortunately, however, there was nothing wrong with Wolgast's hearing. "Wish that fellow would stop calling me crazy," the ex-champion lamented. "It hurts me more than it does him."

One of the physicians turned to the reporters that day and confirmed, "We cannot do anything for him. His mind has lost its grip on all elements of time. Too much battering around the head."

A few weeks later, Judge Robert H. Scott decided that Wolgast, the brilliant future Hall of Famer, could never be released. He was "hopelessly insane."

Wolgast died alone in a blank room in 1955. Punch-drunk syndrome had robbed him of around thirty of his sixty-seven years.

And there were plenty more like him, those whose memories were fast fading, those who were no longer talking as they once had, and those who walked with a stagger in their steps.

* * *

The Marquess of Queensberry Rules, written by Welsh sportsman John Graham Chambers in London in 1865 and published in 1867, were the first guidelines to insist that boxers wear gloves. Bare-knuckle fights under the old London Prize Ring Rules continued for years after, but it was the Marquess of Queensberry Rules that would become more commonplace; by 1889 they were adopted in the United States and Canada.

Among the rules were the terms of battle, which stated that rounds should be three minutes in length with one minute in between; that there could be no wrestling or holding; and that gloves were to be "fair-sized boxing gloves of the best quality and new." These rules formalized the proceedings of combat "to be a fair stand-up boxing match in a twenty-four-foot ring, or as near that size as practicable."

Whether this more polite version of fighting—rather than the bare-knuckle scraps of previous years—was better for fighters is a matter of opinion. There were not many tales of ungloved fighters suffering in retirement, though there were a few. In those days, more battlers suffered from tuberculosis, alcohol consumption, and diabetes as they aged but, of course, punch-drunk syndrome had not been formally identified.

Boxing historian Bob Mee, who wrote the book *Bare Fists* on the pre-gloved era, recognized that some of the heroes of the day developed drinking problems that might have also caused poor health, although Mee conceded that punches may have been a contributory factor. "There were similarities with people who were permanently drunk, who pickled their brains, like Tom Sayers, who had a serious drink problem and was dead at thirty-nine. Now, was that brain damage? We will never know," Mee said.

He continued: "There were people who lived in a complete mess; life expectancy was also shorter in the early days. Were bare-knuckles safer? I don't know. Although those guys obviously took a hell of a lot of punishment, they didn't have as many fights, but the contests they did have were long and arduous. At the same time there was a greater fear of breaking your hand on someone's head, so they punched more sparingly and only when they saw an opening. Those fights we would probably find very boring now. They didn't throw combinations because one false move and you'd break your hand on somebody else's elbow or head, but the principle is the same: you're getting hit on the head and risks would have been there."

Scott Burt runs the Bare Knuckle Boxing Hall of Fame in Belfast, New York. He felt that gloves became a game changer and had been invented to increase knockouts and the volume of punches thrown to make the sport more entertaining.

"People had been leaving many of the bare-knuckle events early because it wasn't exciting and there weren't enough punches," Burt explained. "So the promoters said, 'What can we do to keep people here?' They invented the glove and it made punching more prevalent, not just for training but for actual boxing because then the boxer could whale and whale and whale until a referee—who may or may not have known what he was doing at that time—looked at the guy and somehow magically decided that that guy had had enough. . . . Go over there and punch that wall with your bare fist and you'd tell me I'm stupid. But here, if you put a big pad on your hand, I bet you could hit it a few times."

There was also another side to bare-knuckle fights, Burt added. The media of the time glamorized and exaggerated what violence there was in an attempt to build the gates. "Back then, in the 1880s, they didn't have photographs in the newspapers," he added. "So how were they going to sell more newspapers? They had their artists draw the most gruesome pictures they could of bare-knucklers . . . eyes hanging out . . . teeth all over the place. . . . It was the height of and best example of sensationalism. And the people bought it. Of course they did. They bought the paper; they wanted to see that. They came to the events; they wanted to see that. But the problem is that that image stuck."

* * *

Thus the dangers remained—or were actually increased—once gloves were formally introduced in the sport. And of course, Wolgast was far from the only one showing neurological degeneration or dramatic behavioral alterations. "The Illinois Thunderbolt," Billy Papke, a superb middleweight who as world champion reigned briefly in 1908, killed his wife and then committed suicide in 1936. It has since been suspected that their violent demise came as a result of an undiagnosed dementia and personality change that had been caused by Papke's years of abuse in the ring.

Another middleweight, Kid McCoy, reached his peak around 1906. In 1924, and by then an alcoholic, he was convicted of killing a woman he was seeing. McCoy, paroled in 1932 from San Quentin, took his own life in 1940, leaving a suicide note that simply read: "Sorry I could not endure this world's madness."

And then there were those who just got beaten up and left on the scrap heap to deteriorate. Joe Grim, born Saverio Giannone in Italy in 1881, was renowned for taking endless punishment. Grim prided himself on his ability to take a pounding from the world's top heavyweights and come out unscathed. Those thrashings caught up with Grim, however. Carleton Simon, a psychiatrist and criminologist of the time, attempted to analyze why people knew Joe as "The World's Toughest Man." "Joe Grim is able to stand the terrible beatings to which he has lately been subjected simply owing to the fact that he is in possession of a very small brain," said Simon. "He is of such a low order of intelligence that his nerves, which carry the news to his brain when he is hurt, find a very chilly reception. Now, to grasp the idea that he has been hurt at all, and then not able to take hold of it with one-half the sense of pain of a human being of ordinary intelligence, Grim will have to be almost killed before beaten into insensibility."

Cartoonist and boxing writer Robert Edgren once said of Grim, "Knocking the Iron Man down with fists is a waste of time and effort, for he keeps getting up. To drop Grim for a long count, a boxer—if permitted—should use a crowbar or a baseball bat."

Some three- to five-hundred fights later—by then a serial loser with only a handful of wins—Grim was a wreck. The man newspapers called "The Human Punching Bag" (Grim much preferred "Iron Man") was in an asylum in Byberry near Philadelphia.

Depending on the source, Grim was dead at forty-eight or fifty-three. Broke and neglected, he had evidently not been quite so immune to the effects of the punches that he had taken during his long career after all.

✳ ✳ ✳

While it seemed that there was a limited public awareness of the short-term dangers implicit to the sport of boxing, few if any considered the long-term implications. "They knew that people got damaged but it was kind of accepted," said Bob Mee. "It was kind of acknowledged that that's the cost, that that's what happened. And I don't think people were shocked in the same way. There was the element of 'Oh it will never happen to me,' but there was always the element that 'Well, that's the cost of doing it.' People were looked at with pity if it happened to them, but there was also a shrugging of the shoulders."

As is the case throughout boxing history, only a few were aware of the risks, as well as the clear and present danger. One was respected heavyweight Gene Tunney, who retired as the undefeated world champion in 1928, by coincidence the year that Martland penned "Punch Drunk." It's possible that the well-educated Tunney was aware of the medical journal in question, for after announcing his retirement he told the *New York*

Times on August 3, 1928, why he had decided to retire while arguably still at his peak.

"I went into a clinch with my head down, something I never do," Tunney recalled of one in-ring sparring exchange. "I plunged forward, and my partner's head came up and butted me over the left eye, cutting and dazing me badly. Then . . . he stepped back and swung his right against my jaw with every bit of his power. It landed flush and stiffened me where I stood. . . . That is the last thing I remembered for two days. They tell me that I finished out the round, knocking the man out. From that incident was born my desire to quit the ring forever, the first opportunity that presented itself. . . . But most of all I wanted to leave the game that had threatened my sanity before I met with an accident in a real fight with six-ounce gloves that would permanently hurt my brain."

Later, in his autobiography, Tunney wrote that the possibility of becoming punch-drunk haunted him for weeks.

* * *

Regarding that *Ring* magazine Fight of the Year that opened 1928 with fireworks, Tommy Loughran died on July 7, 1982, at the age of seventy-nine, and Lomski passed away on November 12, 1975, aged seventy-two. They had more than 250 fights between them but later embarked upon different paths. Loughran was one of the great light-heavyweight champions and entered the Marines, becoming a successful sugar broker on Wall Street for more than two decades before stepping down in the 1960s. He had homes in New York and Philadelphia and in retirement spoke at dinners and events promoting the image of boxing and boxers. He had contested an incredible 1,179 rounds of professional fighting.

Lomski turned to wrestling, took on work as a baseball umpire, and was involved in "a few scrapes with the law, not to mention a series of unfortunate auto incidents." In one report, while working as a special police officer in San Francisco, he was arrested for ransacking apartments "looking for papers." The report claimed he stole some items, although the outcome of the incident was not known. The ex-fighter was working as a bouncer at a bar before enlisting in the Merchant Marines. He became a seaman, traveled the world several times, and took work as an engineer on a freighter.

Not everyone was punch-drunk, although the condition adopted many guises. Fighters such as Wolgast had been institutionalized. McCoy had been imprisoned. Papke had simply flipped out. Some, like Ehrlich, toiled in poor health. Others, like Lomski, had experienced spells of erratic behavior while a few, like Loughran, flourished in retirement and grew old gracefully.

Loughran died at the Veterans Home in Hollidaysburg, less than a hundred miles from Pittsburgh. The cause of death, however, remains unknown. There is no evidence with respect to the eventual fate of Lomski or Ehrlich, or the status of their health at the end.

Martland's appeal for deeper research and a greater public awareness of punch-drunk syndrome was largely neglected. That would take many years, and boxing would yield countless casualties.

2

Dementia Pugilistica

A DISEASE THAT
DOESN'T DISCRIMINATE

Gunshots rang out on Aldred Road in Kensington, an upscale area in London. Raymond Henry Bosquet, better known as Canadian middleweight Del Fontaine, and Hilda Meeks were in love—or at least they had been. Then, on the evening of July 10, 1935, at Meeks's mother's house, Fontaine, jealous at a phone call Meeks had received, shot and killed her and injured her mother. He was thirty-one years old; Meeks was just twenty-one.

Fontaine, who had a wife and children back home in Winnipeg, Canada, was a hard puncher but didn't have a sturdy chin. He'd won thirty-seven of fifty-four victories by stoppage or knockout but he'd also been stopped or knocked out fourteen times in his thirty-nine losses. He had turned pro in Canada in 1925, but by 1932 he was fighting almost exclusively in England.

When he was arrested for the shooting, Fontaine said Meeks had broken his heart and ruined his life. However, in a trial that was reported globally, his lawyers presented a different argument: Their main line of defense was that they believed that the boxer was punch-drunk.

Before the court case, Fontaine had apparently confessed to officers: "I shot the girl I really cared for. I don't care if I die. Don't think I'm crazy, boys, because I'm not. She was supposed to be mine but I heard her on the telephone making an appointment for ten o'clock after I would be out. She has ruined my life, home, and children. She had her fortune told by a gypsy who said she would be murdered in three years. I said, 'By God, no,' and I did not think I would be the one to do it. I heard her make the appointment and I shouted in the telephone, 'She's not going to meet you anywhere.' Hilda shouted, 'Yes, I will.' I told her she was going to stay with me. Then her mother came into the room, I said to Hilda, 'I'll shoot you before I let you go with anyone else.' Hilda replied, 'You would not do that.'"

But he did.

In court, friends and other fighters tried to defend Fontaine, saying that after ninety-eight hard fights he was punch-drunk and not of sound mind since losing twelve of his final fourteen fights. Among the witnesses was one of the greats, Ted "Kid" Lewis, who argued Fontaine had taken more punishment than anyone else he'd seen in his time in boxing. "Del shouldn't have been in the ring at all for his last fight," said Lewis. "He wasn't in a fit state."

Boxing manager David Edgar also talked of Fontaine's depleted condition while others spoke of his depressive tendencies. Meanwhile, a doctor's report had found that Fontaine was punch-drunk (although there was no sign of insanity, which his defense had pleaded). Neither the petitions nor protests that called for Fontaine's freedom were successful. On the morning of October 29, 1935, Del Fontaine walked out to the hangman's noose where he was hung in front of a large crowd that had gathered outside Wandsworth Prison. "He was the bravest fellow we ever saw go to the scaffold," said one of the wardens.

* * *

Meanwhile, while Ad Wolgast was struggling in a parallel universe as an ex-champion with punch-drunk syndrome, others were crumbling, shells of once-fit and ambitious young men, now degenerating into frail, fragile, broken shadows. Relics where legends had once been.

Punch-drunk.

Punch-drunk was, of course, the result of repeated blows to the head. How many? It was not known. Over what period of time? It could not be determined. Suffered in the most part by who? No one knew.

But there was a clinical term—encephalopathy—for people who had absorbed numerous blows to the cranium. In 1927, Michael Osnato and Vincent Giliberti had first theorized that "chronic neurodegeneration" could occur even after mild brain trauma. In a hundred cases they discovered that some concussions (in this instance, a blow to the head that had resulted in loss of consciousness "with or without post-traumatic amnesia or skull fracture") resulted in symptoms that continued after the initial impact while others caused degenerative changes. *Traumatic encephalopathy* was defined as a progressive disease found in the brains of people who had taken hits to the head. Encephalopathy came from the Ancient Greek language and could crudely be translated as "brain suffering."

Harrison Martland's pioneering work in "Punch Drunk" had come next. A stand-alone 1929 editorial in the *Journal of the American Medical Association* had agreed that more work was required, saying that Martland's research "resulted in much favorable comment. . . . But a new era in our knowledge of this subject is bound to begin with accurate investigation of the brains thus affected, of the early and late changes, and especially of their topographic distribution."

Research followed from Ernst Jokl in 1933. Then, Harry L. Parker, who was working at the Mayo Clinic in Rochester, Minnesota, wrote the 1934 medical paper "Traumatic Encephalopathy" ("Punch Drunk") of professional pugilists. And in 1936, Martland's assistant, Edward Carroll, surmised that 5 percent of fighters who were in the sport five years or longer would physically suffer, but that around 60 percent from the same time frame would wind up with psychological and emotional changes.

Despite the mounting evidence, everyone went about their business. Risks were ignored and acknowledged in equal measure. It was the price a fighter paid, the chance he took, that he could end up in poor health.

There were still quips about old fighters being punchy, like 1920s middleweight journeyman Frank "The Destroyer" Carbone, a loser in twenty-two of fifty-eight fights, who was spotted outside New York's Roxy Theater shouting at the top of his voice, "People are trying to take me out to the middle of the ocean, right into the waves!"

The symptoms of encephalopathy went beyond physical appearance. Personality changes, depression, suicide, poor business decisions—fighters had suffered from all of them. They always had. Was it because they came from nothing, had nothing, and knew no better, or was it because over the years they had been damaged? In what part was it attributable to their socioeconomics, their backgrounds? And to what extent was it trauma to the head?

Parker, who naturally referenced Martland, used three case studies as he dug for more information. He admitted that, even in 1934, he was writing about "the extremely complicated and highly controversial subject of head injury." He reckoned there were two types: injuries sustained in a fight that might cause death (instantly or within hours), "and those which more by their repetition than by their severity lead to slower development of disability during the fighter's career."

In 1933 the National Boxing Association of America had looked over proposals to introduce leather helmets to prevent punch-drunkenness, an idea that was met with some scorn. A comment piece in *Boxing* magazine referred to the equipment as "a stunt." There are pictures, however, of leather helmets being used in sparring that predate this time. And despite its stance on helmets, *Boxing* agreed that punch-drunkenness wasn't something to dismiss entirely. "I could name many boxers who have been punch-drunk—who have become nervous and physical wrecks—and that is not the thing we want in boxing," read the editorial.

Parker concurred with Martland that "less-expert fighters" were more prone to damage, believing the condition was less common among those who were either more capable defensively or able to finish their opponents quickly, before they could get hit. Parker wrote: "Quick, agile, clever boxers who guard themselves well and take little punishment seem to escape."

Conversely, Parker argued that crowd-pleasers, those who engaged in dramatic slugfests, were more susceptible (which may seem obvious but was pioneering at the time). He had, therefore, been the first man to look at fighting styles and attempt to link them to impairments. "Aggressive, hardy fighters who like to give the crowd an exhibition of blows, and who lead the fight to the end, are likely to suffer," he surmised.

Of course, the term *punch-drunk* was not flattering. Far from it. In fact, it was used in a lawsuit in Britain in the 1930s when it took on libelous implications. In 1939, fight manager Ted Broadribb had sued the *Sunday*

Dispatch and won after the paper had claimed he was punch-drunk. A year before the *Daily Mirror* featured "the scandal of punch-drunk boxers," which claimed that a young boxer, who was managed by his father, had become punch-drunk by taking matches against more-experienced opponents early in his career. The father and son sued the paper; during the trial, the British Boxing Board of Control secretary Charles Donmall said allegations of a punch-drunk fighter indicated "he was so helpless and so battered to pieces that it was impossible for him to engage in a professional boxing contest again." The boxer and his father argued that such bad press meant no promoter would put him on their shows—and they won the case.

In his own research, Parker made it clear that he was trying to analyze the long-term effects of traumatic encephalopathy. He acknowledged Martland's explanation of symptoms—the dragging of one leg or both, tremors, deafness, mental deterioration, and memory loss—and wrote, "It is thus possible that a pugilist may be only mildly affected, and may continue to fight to the end of his career, or he may be so disabled that he ultimately has to quit boxing and yet gets no worse in life. Lastly, a progressive neurological syndrome may appear, putting an end to all fighting, and leading finally to mental or physical helplessness."

There was a pattern, though, that repeated blows to the head compromised the central nervous system.

Of Parker's three cases, the first was a twenty-four-year-old ex-fighter who visited the Mayo Clinic in 1934 because his legs felt weak and his hands shook. He had a flat nose and cauliflower ears, and had retired when he was told he would not make it to the top. He made a comeback, which was as unsuccessful as his first spell. "He was not a very good boxer, although he was willing to take considerable punishment in the hope of getting a final victory by knocking out his opponent or wearing him down. . . . The patient usually made little effort to guard himself," Parker wrote.

He concluded that the beating his case-study patient took on his return to the ring "was responsible for the chain of circumstances that followed." The fighter's brain had been injured, and he never fully recovered.

Parker's second case concerned a thirty-year-old lightweight who first came to him in 1928, experiencing trouble walking and talking. A professional fighter from 1914—when he was sixteen—up to 1921, he was "a second-rate boxer" who often had to show heart and bravery while coming under heavy fire. He was beset by a series of ailments in retirement. Walking was a challenge. His voice became nasal. He was released from working at a mill because of his failing health and by 1923 his right arm was becoming rigid. When he walked "he felt a tendency to be pulled backward." There were headaches, sometimes lasting up to four hours. His memory was impaired and his attention and concentration spans were shorter. He struggled in the six years following his first examination, although the study determined that "he still was able to walk alone, and he could feed and dress himself."

Unlike Parker's Case 1, when a man had returned for a heavy beating and was clearly affected from then on, this case was different. The link between cause and effect was less evident. "All that is known is that after seven years of strenuous fighting and during the course of his career, between one bout and the next, symptoms appeared insidiously, increased in severity, and put an end to his fighting," Parker wrote. "Even after he had left the ring and had tried other pursuits, his difficulties increased steadily up to the time he appeared at the clinic, seven years after his last fight."

Parker's third case looked at a twenty-eight-year-old who initially visited the clinic in 1923, dragging his legs, slurring his words, and with his upper body swaying. A professional for ten years who had fought regularly, he had sometimes boxed as much as three times a week, five times a month, or twenty-two times in a year. He worked as a waiter but tremors meant he would often spill drinks and one day friends began to tease him—"a high grade pugilist"—as "his left leg hit the ground with a slapping noise." It was then he realized things were not right. As his speech thickened and he staggered more frequently in the street, he was often accused of being drunk. His left shoe was worn away where it dragged. Over the next four years, his body became stiff and his movement slowed. As he boxed on he would start fights slowly, move awkwardly, and then loosen into a contest. The disease, however, advanced; and as they say in boxing "caused him to grow old overnight."

"He had been pitted against a boxer whom he easily had beaten before and had expected to beat again," wrote Parker. "In the first few seconds of the first round, while still stiff and awkward, he was given a slight push, stumbled and fell, and was unable even to get back on his feet again. While the crowd howled in derision, his seconds threw in the towel and his last fight was over."

The patient had never been knocked out and said he had never really felt his opponent's blows, despite being a come-forward fighter. Hopes were not high for him and he vanished, seemingly doomed, only for the clinic to write to him some eleven years later in 1934 to discover that "time had dealt gently with him. He seemed in no way worse." The deterioration had inexplicably plateaued rather than progressed. "He had been engaged in various occupations, mainly sedentary, had been moderately successful, and seemed at peace with the world."

Before closing, Parker referred to Ernst Jokl's work and how they had identified three types of injury to the central nervous system that fighters could suffer from: those from a contest, those in the hours and days post-fight, and those later in life. They divided the latter into two categories, physical and mental deterioration.

Parker's three cases formed a complex picture with no exact pattern, only that "scattered lesions of the brain [were] affecting different systems at one and the same time." Yet Parker believed the common denominator was boxing. "The frequency of occurrence of conditions of this kind as reported by others among people who followed the profession of pugilism makes it seem very likely that their profession led to their ultimate disablement," he wrote. He hoped more studies would be forthcoming, leading to more data to support his theories.

✳ ✳ ✳

The work of Parker and Jokl bridged the gap from when "punch-drunk syndrome" became "dementia pugilistica." In fact, Jokl would regularly venture into the territory that was being given a wide berth, by boxing, the medical profession, and in general. Born in Poland, Dr. Ernst Jokl was a founding father of sports medicine in Germany, South Africa, and then the United States, when he moved to Kentucky in the 1950s. In Germany, as a Jew in the 1920s, Jokl was dismissed from his role as the director of the Institute of Sports Medicine in Berlin and he and his wife moved to South Africa where he helped form a national physical-education curriculum for the school system. There he wrote *The Medical Aspect of Boxing*, looking at the sport from hand injuries to concussion and from cauliflower ears to knockouts. He also explored chronic illnesses, such as punch-drunk syndrome. In 1952, his medical work led him to the

United States, where he was one of the eleven founding members of the American College of Sports Medicine (ACSM). In 1993, a high-profile medical award was named after him, the Dr. Ernst Jokl Sports Medicine award. It was first won by a neurologist, Roger Bannister. In 2009 it was won by concussion expert Robert Cantu and in 2016 by pathologist Bennet Omalu, whose research on American football was said to have triggered the NFL's concussion crisis.

Jokl had turned his attention to boxing in the early 1930s as he worked to make "the first comprehensive investigation of the neurological and psychiatric aspects peculiar to boxing." Together with assistant E. Guttman, they examined hundreds of boxers, went to fights, interviewed participants and trainers, studied injured and ill fighters, and performed autopsies on boxers who had died in the ring. Their immediate results were twofold: that there were "immediate effects" and then a "remote sequelae [aftereffects]."

Jokl managed to infiltrate the ranks of boxing people to gain an understanding of the culture. "Head injuries are seldom taken seriously by boxers," he wrote. "Their frequent occurrence leads them to believe that they are of a harmless nature." This brought him to a story from former heavyweight champion Max Baer who, fearful of the left hook of future opponent giant Primo Carnera, asked sparring partners to blast his unguarded jaw with left hooks to toughen him up for the Italian giant. Swedish neurologist Herbert Olivecrona, quoted by Jokl, said of that preparation, "To the question [of] whether one can develop his resisting power in such a way, that one becomes hardened to such blows, the answer is—never! [The brain] cannot be trained for this purpose, and, for heaven's sake, one should never try such an experiment."

Jokl's research went far and wide, and in 1937 he hoped discussions proposing a home for punch-drunk fighters at a National Boxing Association of America convention, which "controlled" boxing in thirty-eight states, would come to fruition. The home would be funded by a levy on all gate receipts at live boxing events. Jokl had high hopes for the place, that not only would it become a sanctuary for retired boxers but a haven for neurologists, where more studies could be carried out. This never happened, of course. Boxing shrugged its shoulders as it always has.

Jokl, who also remarked that a medical professional had made a comment that punch-drunkenness also occurred in football players, was becoming familiar with boxing in all of its grimness and its mechaniza-tions. "Unfortunately, it is true that many, if not the majority of boxers who become punch-drunk are at least in the initial phases of their disease, either unaware of the fact, or, if they are aware of it, continue fighting, mostly for economic reasons until their performances become so weak that they cease to be drawing cards even for a third-rate promoter," he observed. "Some continue to fight as sparring partners, thus receiving further punishment, which will aggravate the harm already suffered by their nervous systems."

In *The Medical Aspect of Boxing*, Jokl explored possible long-term consequences of life in the hardest game, and he became a leading author-ity on boxing injuries. He discussed a "groggy state," describing it as "a degree of cloudiness of the consciousness which leaves intact the auto-matic motoric functions, but interferes with the conception ability, and decreases the reaction rate."

Some of his work mentioned the morality of boxing, not just the sci-ence. "[O]f all major sports, boxing occupies a special position since its aim is that of producing injuries, more particularly to the brain. As the more dramatic manifestations of such injuries are colloquially referred to by such terms as 'knockout,' 'grogginess,' 'punch-drunk,' etc., it is not usually appreciated that similar injuries occur in sports other than boxing, e.g., in football or wrestling. But here they are accidents rather than sequalae of intentional acts. Only in boxing are traumatic injuries unavoidable even if the rules are adhered to."

Jokl retired in 1976, having spent a long time as professor of neurol-ogy and sports medicine at the University of Kentucky.

✸ ✸ ✸

In 1934, the same year that Parker documented his concerns about the sport, a fifty-year-old ex-champion fell to his death from an apartment window deep in a Los Angeles ghetto. Aaron Lister Brown—known as the "Dixie Kid"—had fought some 130 contests between his debut in 1900 and his last bout in 1920. In 1904 he challenged Barbados Joe Walcott for the welterweight title and was losing widely until Walcott was inexplica-bly disqualified in round twenty. (It turned out that the referee had bet on Dixie, and raised his hand. The result was later overturned.) Dixie fought at a high level throughout his career but it wound down in Europe as the inevitable decline set in. By 1922, with his fighting days behind him, he was making loose change playing drums in Berlin and he had hopes of opening a gym. Times were hard. He scrounged for work and asked for handouts until, on April 6, 1934, back in Los Angeles, he plummeted to his death.

Another boxer who did not fare well was world bantamweight and featherweight champion "Terrible" Terry McGovern. Born in 1880, he was a relentlessly aggressive fighter who packed power in both hands. However, after a career of bloody battles that saw him venture up to lightweight where he took on and beat bigger men, he found himself in a life after boxing in which he made bad decisions and both his fortune and his health eroded. McGovern tried to make a comeback—as most fighters do—but the *Montreal Gazette* reported that he was "a shadow of the splendidly developed, sinewy youth who thumped George Dixon into retirement." McGovern was soon finding odd jobs to make money but was also in and out of institutions where doctors tried to discover what was wrong with his rattled brain and addled mind. The ex-boxer fell ill in New York and was admitted to the charity ward of Kings County Hospital in Brooklyn—a mental institute. He died of pneumonia and complications to his kidneys, but his years of fighting, drinking, and yo-yoing from asylum to asylum had not helped. It was a terrible end for "Terrible" Terry. He was only thirty-eight years old.

Another boxer who had symptoms of punch-drunk syndrome later in life was Battling Nelson, nicknamed "the Durable Dane" for his toughness in the ring.[1] In a notorious 1902 war, Nelson traded fifty-one knockdowns with Christy Williams in Arkansas. Williams was down forty-two times before losing in the seventeenth round. Four years later, in September 1906, came one of the sport's infamously controversial bouts, when Nelson boxed Joe Gans. Today, a plaque marks the spot of the marathon fight in the old mining town of Goldfield, Nevada. In the sweltering sun, Nelson forced the pace, attempting to nullify Gans's superior skills. At one point Gans—one of the great lightweights—threw his head between the ropes to vomit. The fight continued, and after twenty rounds Gans was ahead. Nelson, his face a bloody mask, lips severed, peering through slits, was dropped in rounds eight and fifteen, yet he was just getting warm. By the forty-one-round mark, Gans was spent, and as he drunkenly staggered around in the forty-second round, Nelson sought to land the finishing punch. They were in close quarters when, on the referee's blind side, Nelson buried a left hand that caused Gans to crumple to his knees. It looked like Gans might break in half from the body shot, but rather than raise Nelson's arm, the official disqualified Nelson, proclaiming the blow illegal. After two hours and fifty minutes, the longest bout under boxing's new rules, Gans had won on a foul.

Nelson seethed but he would have his revenge two years later, knocking Joe out in seventeen, and three months after that he finished him again in twenty-one rounds.

Two years and eighty hard rounds between them.

In 1909 Nelson lost to Ad Wolgast but a year later they fought a rematch in front of 18,000 people in Richmond, California. The old rivals shared a brutal war until Wolgast ground Nelson to a halt and referee Edward W. Smith rescued a prone Nelson in round forty. It had been scheduled for forty-five.

Ringside reporter, Richard S. Davis, who would later win a Pulitzer for the *Milwaukee Journal*, recalled the gory spectacle with lines such as "Nelson took punch after punch in the face and ribs until he looked like a great chunk of round steak down as far as the belt" and that whenever Wolgast hit him it seemed as though "it was almost like a child pushing his fists into a moist mud pie." In the New York *Herald Tribune*, W. O. McGeehan wrote, "For concentrated viciousness . . . [it was] the most savage bout I have ever seen."

As the astonishing career punishment accumulated, some wanted Nelson to call it a day. "You just can't quit, that's all," the boxer would reply. "They say a criminal is drawn back irresistibly to the scene of his crime. Well, so is a fighter drawn back to the old rings, to the old crowds and to the old excitement."

Nelson fought on. Eighteen times in 1911. Eleven times in 1912.

In 1913, he lost to Wolgast again but nevertheless took fights in Mexico and Cuba before eventually admitting it was over in 1917.

His decline out of the ring was merciless. Nelson made it to the age of seventy-one but "was found to not have his faculties," and Judge Walter J. Stevens committed him to the State Hospital in Illinois. He died in 1954. One obituary—citing officials at the Chicago State Hospital where he had spent his last month—announced "senility" as the cause of death.

* * *

Yet things were changing, gradually. Wheels were turning.

Of course, as Nazi forces grew and spread through Europe, there were more important things in the world in 1937 than the question of who held the heavyweight title. However, almost a decade had gone by since Martland's "Punch Drunk" paper and not a great deal had been done.

Yet while Martland recorded some uncomfortable truths in his groundbreaking research, his naming of the illness as "punch-drunk syndrome" did not sit quite so well with other medical professionals, even if his efforts had. In 1937, writing in the *United States Naval Medical Bulletin*, J. A. Millspaugh sought to change the name of the ailment from "punch-drunk syndrome" to "dementia pugilistica." He felt the name "punch-drunk syndrome" was condescending, that afflicted fighters were probably lesser boxers—as Martland and Parker had assumed—and that the name itself was in no way flattering, even though he had witnessed behavioral similarities between old fighters and drunks. "Punch drunk implies a derisive connotation, especially among collegiates; even the hardened professional resents the implication," assessed Millspaugh. "The most typical examples of this disorder are usually found among the less expert boxers, particularly as concerns defensive ingenuity."

Through his experiences of the disease, Millspaugh was aware of exactly why negative connotations might follow. "I have known an ex-fighter to be considered as inebriated by ward mates when he had not a swallow of intoxicant over a long period," Millspaugh explained. "The heavy, mouthy 'set' voice, jerky, sluggish movement together with the subjective symptoms of daze just short of mild vertigo, combined to produce this impression."

Millspaugh conferred with colleagues, "several naval medical officers," and—with just one exception—they agreed "that there are definite neurological, intellectual, and personality changes presented by typical fighters, particularly those of the older order who fought more often, certainly longer and perhaps harder."

In recording the signs of dementia pugilistica, Millspaugh concentrated first on appearances, citing swollen ears, flattened noses, and scar tissue around the eyes. He wrote that some fighters possessed an inability to speak, caused by battered larynxes, as well as broken noses and teeth that could make voices "hoarse, rasping, coarse, or thick" following "an alteration of both primary and secondary speech channels." The difficulty in walking, known as dysbasia, was monitored as Millspaugh observed "swaying, shuffling, staggering, and later a propulsive or festinating gait." Then there were periods of amnesia.

As well as the physical toll fighting was taking on the boxers, there were further costs, including erratic behavior and tragic early deaths.

With an almost lighthearted look at the condition, Millspaugh wrote about an observation he had made that demonstrated behavioral changes and illustrated how the illness was being dismissed. "One morning while awaiting a boat aboard a cruiser I was attracted by the unusual behavior of the officer of the deck," Millspaugh wrote. "Judging by his boisterous activity (vocal, pantomime, and footwork) one might envisage him directing a deadly engagement, the outcome of which was by no means certain. Inquiry revealed he was a well-known athlete while at the Naval Academy. Over a year later I had the occasion to see him burst into a room where five medical officers were temporarily assembled. He chose a seat on the windowsill, spouted forth concerning his ailment, and abruptly departed in a dash. Upon his departure the doctors variously shook their heads, lightly smiled, regarded another with questioning gaze, and one murmured, 'punch-drunk.'"

Shoulders were shrugged and they went about their business.

In his paper, Millspaugh became entwined in a moral conflict. He felt that many managers overmatched inexperienced fighters or that sometimes boxers who had not been in training were bought in and served up to opponents—for money. He pondered, "Why are fighters invariably associated with managers who in most instances conserve more gain than their charges, few of whom retain any considerable material resources? It may be objected that fighters as a class do not stand high mentally but certainly as high as many other groups who fare better in after years." He sympathized with boxers. "Indeed, some escape the most and worst but few, if any, escape all the signs and symptoms."

Millspaugh had made his summaries based on years of watching fights and fighters. He had not presented any detailed analysis of case studies but had witnessed "many individuals" who suffered.

"A new term is proposed for a condition long recognized but accorded little medical cognizance," he declared. While the name was seemingly still up for debate, the symptoms were not and Millspaugh proposed that "dementia pugilistica" was a much more acceptable and palatable term than punch-drunk-syndrome. He, as Martland had before him, seemed to imply that more studies would follow. But with the world on the brink of war, the priority was not old fighters slurring their words or walking on their heels.

* * *

Regardless of what anyone chose to call it, there was a grave acceptance that boxing was Russian roulette with gloves. You start taking the punches and slowly the chamber empties. The wider concern was what happened with one fatal shot, but these medical pioneers were equally anxious about the cumulative effects of waiting for the bullets to fire. What was happening shot after shot to the man on the receiving end day after day in the gym and fight after fight in the prize ring?

Pockets of research were being conducted at a similar time. In 1937 C. E. Winterstein wrote "Head Injuries Attributable to Boxing" in *The Lancet*. He said boxers winding up punch-drunk was because of "continued hammering."

Three years later Karl Mudock Bowman and Abram Blau wrote "Psychotic States Following Head and Brain Injury in Adults and Children."

They were brought to the subject while investigating compensation claims in the aftermath of traffic accidents. They were seeing whether long-term brain disease was a reason for the accidents, speculating that potential claimants might have been suffering from "traumatic encephalopathy of pugilists or punch-drunk."

Bowman and Blau went over previously trodden ground, claiming only fighters who were not very good were at risk. However, they did say that the boxers would be the last to realize that they had been damaged, adding that those around them, be it family or management, would be able to see the symptoms first.

The scientists actually visited a psychiatric division of a hospital to examine an old fighter, diagnosing "chronic traumatic encephalopathy of pugilists" and it was quite possibly the first time that the term and the sport had been linked.

* * *

Thus, in 1937, "punch-drunk syndrome" gave way to "dementia pugilistica." It was not just old fighters who suffered from it. Nor, as the early research showed, was it just novices, sparring partners, and fall guys. Some fighters were burnt out before others, some fought long, hard careers, some were "punchy" after a dozen fights. There was no set pattern but there was plenty of coincidence.

Boxing's highfliers back then had been Joe Louis, Sugar Ray Robinson, and Henry Armstrong. All three would battle dementia pugilistica as they grew old.

Louis had been a straight shooter who, in retirement from boxing, enjoyed golf and dressed smartly. But his wife at the time, Martha, began to note behavioral changes. Sometimes he would go days without changing his clothes. The golfing stopped. He became reclusive. Paranoia started to set in and he feared the Mafia was out to kill him. As his psychological problems took hold, Louis was hospitalized in Colorado. His family did not say much and the press sympathized with his plight.

Initially, doctors reported that boxing had not caused damage to his brain and Louis saw a psychiatrist. He returned to Las Vegas to work as a greeter in Caesars Palace and enjoyed doing it, even if others felt it was a demeaning way for an old icon to make a buck. When he relapsed and his wife intervened to put him in an institution for his own well-being, Louis believed the Mob was behind it.

Louis stopped a coke habit in his fifties but still smoked and boozed. His behavior remained inconsistent. In October 1977 he had a massive heart attack and a cerebral hemorrhage. It left him confined to a wheelchair and he had trouble speaking.

Four years later, in April 1981, he went to watch Larry Holmes defeat Trevor Berbick for his old heavyweight title at Caesars and died at home the next morning from another heart attack. An obituary of the legend in a Des Moines newspaper read, "He was a gentleman, a great fighter, and in his later years a pathetic figure."

He wasn't the only one.

Fellow 1930s legend "Homicide Hank," as Henry Armstrong was known, went from running a nightclub in Harlem—the Melody Room—to becoming a born-again Christian and an ordained minister. He taught youngsters how to fight, too.

The only boxer to hold three world titles in three weight classes (featherweight, lightweight, and welterweight) at the same time, Armstrong died of heart failure after a long series of illnesses, including—according to his *New York Times* obituary—pneumonia, cataracts, anemia, malnutrition, and dementia. He had fought more than 180 times from 1931 to 1945, but it was after taking a beating in the streets in his old St. Louis neighborhood that his decline in health triggered and possibly accelerated the dementia. Thieves stole the then sixty-nine-year-old ex-fighter's wallet and Hall of Fame ring, and all he could say in the hospital was, "I would have taken them both out in a minute in my prime."

As the years rolled on mercilessly, Armstrong needed someone to shave and wash him and to help him get dressed. When he died in October 1988, in a hospital bed at age seventy-eight, he was virtually blind and his body had decayed to only a hundred pounds.

During his final years, his wife Gussie had looked after the boxing superstar. "I do what I can for him," she said. "But it's like the song. Nobody wants you when you're down and out."

His welterweight rival, Sugar Ray Robinson, was also struggling. When Robinson was in his fifties, his family started to notice changes. He'd started a youth foundation in California but Katy Riny, who was on the staff there, said he was developing nervous habits, his speech was becoming slurred, and he was slowing down. Some thought he'd started to smoke marijuana as he was becoming more paranoid and he was actually diagnosed with premature senility. Dave Anderson, who wrote Robinson's autobiography with the legend, recalled their meetings as Ray reached the end. "He would sit there looking straight ahead and [his wife] Milly would bend down to him and say, 'Ray, Ray, Dave Anderson's here. It's Dave. Say hi.' And his face would brighten, he'd stand up, shake hands, give you a little hug, and then he would sit back down and go right into that glazed look."

Visitors said that when he could no longer talk, there was a "sort of a droning sound coming from his throat."

Hearing he was in poor health, friends flew from New York to California, where he'd moved, but he didn't recognize them. At a benefit in his honor, old foes lined up to greet him. He didn't recognize Gene Fullmer, whom he'd fought four times.

"It wasn't so much sad as it was revealing about life, fighters, this was the greatest fist fighter that ever lived, so if this is what happened to him, this is what happens to them all," said the late sportswriter Ralph Wiley.

3

A Slick Medical Cliché

DENIERS AND
DOUBTERS OF CTE

There was "a wino derelict along New York's Tenth Avenue," wrote the city's *Police Gazette* in 1961.

Twenty years earlier, Herbert Lewis Hardwick, also known as Cocoa Kid, was a fighting terror, avoided by the very best of his era, trapped in a vortex with half a dozen other hard-luck, hard-done-by fighters from lightweight to light heavyweight. They could not get championship shots because they were either too good, too black, or they were not well-connected.

But in 1961, Cocoa Kid was broke, homeless, and physically and mentally ruined. He could hardly talk as he traipsed Manhattan for handouts. He was severely punch-drunk.

Hardwick was born in Puerto Rico in 1914 and boxed some 250 times as a professional.[2] He was a terrific welterweight and middleweight who longed to fight Henry Armstrong and Sugar Ray Robinson but never did. He was part of what was called the Murderers' Row, a rough, talented, and uncompromising batch of contenders and gatekeepers forced to earn their living on the peripheries of the biggest fights. They ended up fighting each other. A lot. Charley Burley was the best of the bunch but Cocoa Kid, Holman Williams, Lloyd Marshall, Jack Chase, Eddie Booker, Aaron Wade, and Bert Lytell were a problem for anybody. They were definitely a problem for one another. Cocoa Kid fought Burley twice, Williams thirteen times, and Chase, Wade, and Lytell each three times. The chances are they battered themselves into a horrid oblivion waiting for a door to open without even being able to force it ajar.

Kid just could not get a shot. At welterweight he chased Henry Armstrong and at middleweight he pursued Sugar Ray Robinson. Despite several long unbeaten runs in the late 1930s and early 1940s, neither fight materialized.

In 1943, having turned pro in 1929 and racking up dozens of professional contests, Kid was enlisted into the Naval Reserves but was promptly discharged, returning to the only thing he knew: the prize ring. He fought about forty more bouts but was already damaged goods and deteriorating. We know this because the Navy discharged him on medical grounds. "Dementia pugilistica" was listed on his file. It was not a common prognosis of the day. Perhaps the doctors in the services, knowing his profession, had read J. A. Millspaugh's medical work in the *Navy Bulletin*.

As Kid boxed on, he kept his ailments under wraps as best as he could, sparring and fighting hundreds upon hundreds more damaging rounds. He even reportedly once floored Sugar Ray Robinson in a training session, but he never got his title shot.

His last recorded outing was against Bobby Mann, a decent local fighter in Trenton, New Jersey. Kid lost, as they mostly all do in their farewells. It was a timid defeat over eight rounds. The year was 1948 and he had been fighting relentlessly for two decades.

By 1959, Kid was lost in a demented world. Boxing writer Springs Toledo brought those sad days to life: "He wasn't sure of his name anymore, this tattered figure wandering Times Square. 'Heriberto Harwit' was as close as he could get [in his attempts to say Herbert Hardwick]. . . . He'd shuffle over to the general delivery window at 33rd and 8th and mumble to the clerk. His VA [Veterans Affairs] benefit check was his only income, but he'd often lose his service papers and had to find a way to the local veterans' office and fill out an application for copies. Staff had a fine time trying to sort through the misinformation he provided—he forgot where and when he was born. 'January 9, 1916, in Mexico' he guessed on one application. He was actually born on May 2, 1914, in Puerto Rico."

It got worse for Kid. Living off benefits he somehow found his way into Chicago's Dunning Asylum. No one knew who he was. Neither did he. It was only when they matched his fingerprints to his Naval records that they found out.

* * *

MacDonald Critchley was born in 1900. A dashing English gentleman, he was a behavioral neurologist. Educated in Bristol, in the west of England, he moved to London where he worked at the King's College Hospital on Queen's Square. After a series of promotions, Critchley became the president of the World Federation of Neurology. In the late 1940s, he began to look at boxing and, specifically, the changes in behavior that fighters experienced during and after their careers. He wrote that he believed that "probably the most important neurological consequence of boxing . . . is the so-called punch-drunk syndrome." He founded the Migraine Trust and wrote a biography on James Parkinson, the English surgeon. Parkinson had written "An Essay on the Shaking Palsy" back in 1817, describing the condition that was later named after him, Parkinson's.

Critchley's early work on boxers was done around the same time J. A. Millspaugh published his thoughts and findings, after he had described long-term damage from boxing as "dementia pugilistica"—but Critchley was still not satisfied with the name. There may have been a moral argument, but clinically the name was not entirely accurate because dementia was not always present, he contended. As there was not a specific set of symptoms, the name for punch-drunk or dementia pugilistica changed often, even if the overall picture of the disease was the same. There were memory problems, signs of dementia, mood changes, and motor skills failing either independently or in combination.

But, in his 1957 *British Medical Journal* paper "Medical Aspects of Boxing, Particularly from a Neurological Standpoint," Critchley was still trying to come up with a different, more fitting term. He preferred "chronic progressive traumatic encephalopathy of boxers." He published findings of sixty-nine fighters suffering from the effects of their careers and discovered that symptoms began to show themselves on average about sixteen years after a fighter had laced up gloves for the first time. The signs progressed and were irreversible.

In 1962, Cyril Brian Courville—"scholar, scientist and artist," according to his *Journal of the American Medical Association* obituary—reckoned "psychopathic deterioration of pugilist" was a better title for the illness. In 1963, G. La Cava suggested the name "cumulative traumatic encephalopathy of the boxer" while C. Mawdsley and F. R. Ferguson, still trying to identify the problems faced by fighters, studied ten cases. One boxer was "liable to have outbursts of rage and violence," but another only began showing symptoms twenty-five years after retiring—though they did not rule out cerebrovascular disease.

Critchley's long, clumsy title—"chronic progressive traumatic encephalopathy of boxers"—described how illness could appear slowly but then progress and develop. Symptoms may even show themselves in retirement, with the boxer apparently unscathed after his last fight. However, Critchley had noted that the more physical alterations a man had endured from fighting, the more chance there was of him suffering down the line. Did he have cauliflower ears? Was his nose battered flat? Was there scar tissue around his eyes? These could be precursors, symbols of damage that had occurred externally with a possible cost neurologically. Critchley also felt the problem was more common in white fighters but, like others before him, he worried for boxers who, simply put, weren't that good.

Critchley, arguably using a sporting mind rather than a medical one, said the telltale signs came when a boxer started to lose contests he was expected to win. Again, there was no set criteria as to which fighters were being affected and how badly. Critchley wrote that some damaged boxers "seem to have a raised threshold, being able to take progressively more and more punishment before going down, while in others the opposite occurs. These latter cases are sometimes called to be 'glassy jaws.'"

"I can't think properly," one boxer told Critchley. "And I can't remember things; my speech has been getting bad for eighteen months. . . . My head goes blank at times."

Another of Critchley's damaged studies was sixty-one years old and fought professionally from 1910 to 1926. He said he would not allow his children to fight. "It ought to be stopped," he felt.

Others displayed memory loss, seizures, tremors, walked unsteadily, and their speech was slurred. Some had been in trouble with the law; one was actually interviewed and examined in prison; others were finding problems with their vision and hearing. One "tended to dribble," another showed "both an intellectual falling-off and a curious alteration in personality," and their fighting powers dimmed as their careers neared the end. One was in such bad shape when he got into the ring to box that "he staggered so much that the audience howled him down and the promoter declared him drunk."

In more than a hundred cases of neurological diseases in boxing, Critchley said the majority should be considered punch-drunk, be it an early diagnosis or with well-established symptoms. He suspected the disease was more prevalent in professionals than amateurs, too.

There were plenty of sweeping statements, but Critchley contended that despite the problem of punch-drunk syndrome being known about for three decades, there had been such little work done that he could be forgiven for blindly trying to find some rhyme or reason for it. "As fighters, the punch-drunk ex-pugilists have been slow on their feet rather than nimble, and notorious as being able to 'take it,'" he said. "They can perhaps be looked upon as 'sluggers' rather than scientific boxers. Punch-drunken states have been found in fighters of all weights, particular about the size of their opponents, having often taken on contestants heavier than themselves."

In England, at carnivals and fairgrounds, fighters used to compete in what were officially known as "boxing booths" but were also referred to as "blood tubs." Those who endured countless battles in them were also at risk, Critchley determined.

Regardless of how a boxer became afflicted with the disease, Critchley noted the following symptoms: a fighter would slow down, he was not overly aware of his own deterioration, the memory went, and there were mood swings and irritability and sometimes uncharacteristically violent behavior. Then there were tremors. Slurred speech. Rigidity.

Of the cases Critchley examined, one had been a sparring partner of heavyweight king Max Baer, another was a super bantamweight who had been knocked out some sixty times, while a twenty-seven-year-old welterweight had been knocked out three times during his career. The latter started losing his temper and began to tremble as he grew older. Eleven of

Critchley's cases showed signs of punch-drunkenness in its various guises and Critchley, in explaining traumatic encephalopathy, added, "Once established it not only does not permit of reversibility, but it ordinarily advances steadily. This is the case even though the boxer has retired from the ring and repeated cranial traumata are at an end."

Critchley wrote that a victim could be affected by symptoms for several days after a fight, suffering from headaches, dizziness, and imbalances. It passes, though, and then the boxer goes back to normal. However, Critchley felt that it always happened at a cost. "The suggestion, indeed, that an accumulation of groggy states leads to a permanent punch-drunken clinical picture is not to be considered far-fetched," he stated.

In his conclusion, he felt more scans of boxers at varying stages of their careers could illustrate a more rounded picture of any condition and that practicing neurologists should look into both the "groggy state" and "the condition known as traumatic progressive encephalopathy (or punch-drunkenness)."

"Owing to the extreme paucity of pathological data, it is highly desirable that opportunity should be afforded neuropathologists of studying the appearances of the brain of punch-drunk patients," Critchley wrote.

*　*　*

By now, and with the 1950s invention of the jet engine taking off, boxing was becoming more worldwide than ever. In Vic Toweel, Jimmy Carruthers, the brilliant Pascual Perez, Hogan "Kid" Bassey, and Yoshio Shirai, South Africa, Australia, Argentina, Nigeria, and Japan celebrated their first world champions respectively. The sport was truly going global while fighters like Rocky Marciano, Archie Moore, Sugar Ray Robinson, Sandy Saddler, and Willie Pep were big news in America.

Incidentally, Carruthers would later suffer with Parkinson's, Bassey with dementia, while Saddler and Pep had Alzheimer's in their old age.

Yet the trade rarely discussed the problem. There is more about it in medical papers of the time than in boxing magazines. An October 1953 article in *The Ring* was headlined, "Demand for Boxers' Insurance Grows," and writer Donald "Ridge" McArthur opined, "No one will deny that bad jokes about 'punch-drunk' fighters have injured the sport's reputation. The disfigured faces of some 'old timers' have certainly prejudiced some parents against permitting talented youngsters to seek boxing careers." He said that those "offensive conditions" had been "substantially eliminated" by "progressive safety steps taken by boxing commissions the country over."

But through the 1940s and 1950s, another fighter was falling into trouble. "Slapsie" Maxie Rosenbloom had been a former world light-heavyweight champion, a veteran of some 298 professional fights, completing a mind-boggling 2,524 rounds. In retirement, he found his way into the entertainment world, acting on TV, radio, and in films. Often he would play the role of a clumsy but lovable punch-drunk fighter, his thick and deteriorating New York accent—"do'es, dem's, dee's"—lent itself to the parts, as did his thick, cauliflowered left ear.

He appeared alongside Marlene Dietrich in *The Fred Allen Show*, was in *Each Dawn I Die,* and had a prominent role in *Requiem for a Heavyweight*. In Rod Serling's hit, *Requiem*, Rosenbloom played a retired pug who told old war stories to other used-up fighters in a dive bar.

But as time went by, friends were concerned that Rosenbloom was no longer playing the fool. He couldn't recognize his pals, would repeat the same story over and over—forgetting he had just told it—and his speech worsened. He could no longer run his LA nightclub, Slapsie Maxie's, and lost everything, living in an asylum in his sixties with his doctor saying too many punches had caused his demise.

Others speculated that his downward spiral only started when he was mugged and hospitalized after leaving a nightclub in 1968, when he was reportedly hit over the head with a pipe. Either way, the degeneration was underway.

Those who loved Rosenbloom—and he was always a popular figure—defended him. Protective relatives and friends staunchly denied that he had actually been punch-drunk. It was deemed embarrassing, not least because scientists continued to implore that it happened to fighters who weren't very good. Rosenbloom was good and defensively he was a bag of tricks. A *Los Angeles Times* column around the time of his death commented, "The doctors said he took too many punches and there was 'a good deal of damage to his brain.' That's got to be a lie. Nobody ever hit Maxie."

A man who Rosenbloom was in the nightclub business with, Sammy Lewis, contended Rosenbloom "went senile, not punchy," before conceding, "If you take those punches, something's got to give."

Rosenbloom tried to maintain his sense of humor as the end neared. He was visited by an old foe from their time boxing in the Pacific during the war in his later years but he didn't recognize him. "Maxie, you remember New Caledonia, don't you?" the man asked, hopefully. Rosenbloom looked back vacantly and replied, "I don't even remember Old Caledonia."

Rosenbloom died in 1976, but for the last four years of his life, the executive director of the Motion Picture Fund had been made his legal guardian after the "alleged incompetent"—then sixty-seven years old— had been sent to the Braewood Sanitarium in South Pasadena.

It was another sad boxing end.

* * *

Around the same time that Rosenbloom was falling ill, New Orleans super welterweight Ralph Dupas was dancing through a wave of contenders. Dupas had what was referred to as a New Orleans style, boasting quick, nimble, fancy footwork that kept him out of harm's way and allowed him to spring forward with rapid-fire attacks. Dupas was no puncher, though, with just 19 stoppage wins in 106 victories against 23 losses and 6 draws. But he was good, a skillful operator who was unfortunate to come up against Joe Brown, Emile Griffith, Sugar Ray Robinson, Del Flanagan, and Florentino Fernandez in a rough and talent-laden era.

But in the long run, Dupas's fancy footwork was turned into a slow, agonizing shuffle. He fought on too long and, as his skills declined, he wound up working in casinos in Las Vegas and was then pushing around shopping carts in Sin City parking lots collecting bottles to sell to pay for his dilapidated rented room. His family brought him back to New Orleans where dementia pugilistica was diagnosed, and he spent years staring blankly at the walls while rocking back and forth. Finally, he was placed in a home in Denham Springs, where he saw out the rest of his empty days. He died at the age of seventy-two in 2008.

There was another Ralph Dupas, a nephew. Pete Dupas named his son after his famous brother, and little Ralph wanted to get into boxing. Pete wouldn't let him after what happened to his sibling so the youngster got into horse racing instead. He was good, won plenty, but once when he fell off he was kicked in the head, the horse landed on him, and he fractured his skull. It was a traumatic, life-changing accident. "We talk about Uncle Ralph sometimes," Pete said, "and you know it's strange. I look at my brother and what boxing did to him. Then I look at my son. My son loved racing the way my brother loved boxing. You just never know."

✳ ✳ ✳

For his book *In This Corner*, author Peter Heller talked to some of the leading fighters from each decade from the 1920s all the way through to the 1970s. He conducted forty-two long-form first-person interviews. Years later, after *In This Corner* was consigned to history, boxing historian Mike Silver came to own more than twenty of the audiotapes that featured the interviews. The likes of Paul Pender, Jack Dempsey, Jimmy McLarnin, Willie Pep, Mickey Walker, Beau Jack, and many more recalled the highs and lows of their careers.

"I have met many, many fighters," said Silver of his half century in the sport. "I've met many punchy fighters and it's awful. You can hear the progression in [their] voice . . . if you listen to Jack Dempsey, who was always in the public eye and was always talking to people, he developed some compensatory behavior, but if you listen to an older Jack Dempsey there's a slight slur in his voice, 'How ya doin' buddy? How ya dooin'?' There's that slur that you hear. I've seen it in fighters who I knew when they first started and then years later they were still okay in their forties and they could function and then something happened. When their brain aged, they had no compensation, they had no ability to try and do anything about it. By their sixties, their memories were going and they were having problems remembering simple things and the shaking of the hands might have started and certainly if they live to seventy, they're pretty much out of it. They need people to take care of them. I've seen it. I've seen other fighters who, as they get older, they began to slur their words, like they'd had a few too many drinks."

Mike Silver started boxing as an amateur at fourteen and had three amateur fights but after one sparring session he was left with a terrible headache. It was so severe it put him off his studies and he made the decision that if he passed his college exams it was time to stop boxing.

Silver, who has been in and around New York gyms since the 1960s where he used to break bread with the likes of Ray Arcel in Stillman's

Gym, noticed a pattern, however: Fighters in their thirties, forties, and fifties were generally okay, and then there was a sad, steep decline.

"Now [Fritzie] Zivic, who had 230-something fights, he developed Alzheimer's," said Silver. "Well, they call it Alzheimer's. He stopped being able to take care of himself in his sixties, I would say, before he fell apart completely and there was no reserve. In this tape of Fritzie Zivic, he's talking about his fights. This was done in 1970 so how old was Fritzie? He was born in 1913 so around fifty-seven. He had that quick way of speaking that the fighters have, you can see that they took too many punches as they speak a little quickly—it's a speech pattern. My ear is very attuned to it because ever since I was a teenager and I got concerned about my own brain damage I would focus on the fighters and hear how their speech patterns were changing. I knew, hearing him speak, that when he gets into his early sixties he's going to be 'gone.' And sure enough, if you read the obituaries of all these fighters. . . ."

Silver continued: "I remember I was in Arizona in 1993 and at the time Lou Ambers [a world lightweight champ] would have been about eighty, and I called up his wife and I said, 'I'm here, I'm a big boxing fan, I'm also a writer, I'd like to meet with Lou.' And she said, 'He doesn't remember anything. You wouldn't get anything out of the interview. Please, there's no point to it.' And I've got that a number of times trying to interview old fighters. However, I have interviewed a number of old fighters who have had forty, fifty fights who are about eighty years old and who exhibited almost no damage. There was a fighter, Ted Lowry [a Massachusetts heavyweight who died at ninety], and when I interviewed him he was eighty-two years old and he had 148 pro fights and he was a journeyman, a very good defensive fighter, and this guy was amazing. If you saw him, you'd say, 'I can't believe this guy ever had a professional fight.' Archie Moore, 216 fights or whatever and he was cogent and clear almost to the day he died. He might have slowed up but he was sharp as a tack. They are exceptions. Maybe it's something genetically, maybe it's a combination of them being good defensively but still their careers were so long. Archie Moore was knocked out seven, eight, nine times. The point is, how come they escaped it? How come there are guys who smoked their entire lives, never got lung cancer? We know them. There are guys who eat terribly and live to their nineties, others drop dead of a heart attack in their forties. So there is an aspect of genetics, a structure of the skull I believe and I'm just theorizing maybe the way their brain was against the skull and there wasn't as much room to jostle, or maybe their necks were just so strong or something that their heads didn't move like another fighter. We just don't know."

* * *

Other boxers from Heller's book were slowly in decline, but it was sometimes tough to distinguish whether the boxers were punch-drunk, whether they had behavioral issues, or whether they had a combination of the two.

Former world welterweight champion Don Jordan was a prime example. He was born in the Dominican Republic in 1934 but moved to the United States and in 1958 he defeated Virgil Akins for the title. By the time he spoke to Heller, he was a divorced recovering alcoholic. He told Heller he had been a paid assassin, at one point killing thirty people in a month. Heller noted that this was not true, but he indulged Jordan who told him of how he'd killed with poisoned bamboo darts to the neck and how the police didn't want to arrest him because they were scared. Jordan claimed he had lived a parallel life. What hadn't helped him was the Mob's tight control in boxing, and he admitted to taking dives at the behest of the gangsters who were running the sport at the time.

Silver doesn't believe that boxing was entirely to blame for Jordan's unraveling. Jordan's rap sheet was possibly longer than his boxing record. He'd been caught with marijuana, was arrested for drunk driving, once fired arrows from a sixty-inch target bow at two women, and, after he was arrested and during questioning, he attempted to reach for the bow to fire it at the officers and journalists who were covering the story. He'd made bad business deals, had gotten involved with the wrong people, had won only two of his last eleven fights, and then was thrown out of the sport by the California State Athletic Commission because they thought he'd taken a dive in his last contest, a meek decision defeat to Raymundo "Battling" Torres. Two years from champion of the world to rock bottom.

"No, I don't think so," said Silver when asked whether Jordan's erratic behavior had been due to punches. "He was a good boxer, never took a severe beating, but a lot of times when a fighter is managed by the Mob, they're given instruction to lose, they're taken advantage of. These fighters realize they have no control over their own careers and they see these guys who are murderers and so on, and they fear them. Was the fact that the paranoia that he had, was that accentuated because of the punches he took? The man was obviously out of his mind. I don't believe any of that stuff, that he said he was a hitman and he had killed about thirty people. He might have ended up in mental institution had he not taken just one punch. We just don't know."

Jordan was robbed and assaulted in a Los Angeles parking lot in 1997 before dying in a home from his injuries. He'd been in a coma for five months and the two men accused of beating him were released due to insufficient evidence.

* * *

Another of Heller's subjects was Emile Griffith, the great former welter-weight and middleweight, who was from a similar era as Jordan.

"Emile Griffith was OK," recalled Silver. "He had brain damage, there's no question about it, but I did an interview with him in 1998, so he was sixty years old and he answered questions and he was talking. . . . [A] neuroscientist friend of mine looked at him and said there's definite brain damage here, but [Griffith] was capable of going up to the Hall of Fame, signing autographs, talking to fans. . . . However, within seven or eight years of that interview he was basically no longer compos mentis."

Griffith was attacked one night outside a nightclub, and that seemed to accelerate his fall into darkness.

* * *

Meanwhile, Critchley was researching boxing's links to long-term brain injuries as well as illnesses including Parkinson's and Alzheimer's. He would write more than twenty books and, as one of the world's leading neurologists, he had more than two hundred articles published on the subject.

Case after case was examined, amateur fighters and professionals, retired and active. There was still a stigma attached to how good a fighter was, in that the bad ones were more at risk of being harmed in the long term as well as the short, scientists believed.

Yet still there were doubters. Harrison Martland had met resistance in 1928 when he spoke to "one sporting writer of note" who, he reported, "has recently stated that punch-drunk was greatly exaggerated and that he had consulted eminent neurologists who assured him that such [a] condition did not exist." That fighters were slurring, staggering, and forgetting to varying degrees was merely circumstantial. That some were making poor decisions in retirement, becoming depressed, splitting from loved ones, and losing fortunes was put down to someone coming from nothing and not knowing how to handle everything.

The dissenters of medicine and science were vocal. Some wanted to protect the sport they loved and some needed it to make a living. They supported boxing, not research. Dementia was not in their best interest. They preferred talking about phantom punches rather than phantom illnesses.

A 1950s UK television documentary called *The Has Beens* looked at retired fighters and what happened to them in life after boxing. Respected reporter Denzil Batchelor narrated and posed difficult questions to several old boxers. Batchelor traced all ten living flyweight and bantamweight British champions from World War I to the end of World War II. Five of the ten had been institutionalized, at least six of them had broken marriages, two had been convicted for acts of violence, and the majority had lost their wealth. Alf Kid Pettenden was a former British bantamweight champion who ended up living on assistance in Tottenham having suffered a "breakdown in health." Tommy Noble, another old British bantamweight champ, wound up in a mental hospital, as did Bugler Harry Lake, whose condition was so severe that the film crews were neither allowed to interview nor picture him.

Yet some of the men denied that their ailments were caused by boxing. Former British flyweight champion Jackie Brown thought that the way he walked with a lurch was caused by arthritis. Journeyman featherweight Jackie Chambers thought he slurred because he'd had a new set of false teeth put in. The great Jimmy Wilde thought his memory was just fine, even as he shuffled around at the age of seventy-three.

"How many fights did you have? Do you know?" asked Batchelor.

"I know all right," Wilde snapped. "I had about . . . about 100, I think."

It's been recorded as 142.

"You don't remember very well?" Batchelor pressed.

"No, I don't. If I did, I would be on top of the world now."

But both Brown and Chambers were partially aware of the changes that had occurred. "I've got a damaged brain, a very damaged brain," muttered Brown, who said he'd ban the sport with what he'd learned about it. "It doesn't affect my walking, my walking's affected by arthritis, not by fighting, by arthritis, but it affects my speech very bad."

Chambers, interviewed in a psychiatric unit, said he could feel himself slowing down at the age of thirty-nine and that throughout his career he'd been too brave for his own good. "I should have laid down as I'd have felt better now and I would have felt better in my brain," he said.

Then the denial kicked in, as it often did. "I definitely think I'm not [punch-drunk]," Chambers added, answering the direct question from Batchelor. "I'm not punchy, but it so happens that I have taken unnecessary punishment in the ring."

Some say Wilde was Britain's greatest-ever fighter. He became a boxing writer but found himself being cared for when he could no longer do it himself.

"If you were a young man, would you become a boxer?" Batchelor asked him.

"Yes, I would," Wilde replied.

"Why?"

"Well, I love it."

All in all, it was a damning film but there were plenty who turned a blind eye.

Wilde died in 1968. Author Peter McInness, writing in an updated version of Wilde's autobiography *Fighting Was My Business*, wrote a stirring farewell to the great "Mighty Atom": "He became bed-ridden and he never did come to realize that his dear wife, Elizabeth, had died nearly two years earlier. Happily, the hospital nurses loved him and one of them, young enough to have been his grandchild, said that he looked more like an innocent young child rather than a once-great professional pugilist as the end drew nigh."

Meanwhile, Batchelor claimed that the British Boxing Board of Control had told him punch-drunkenness was "almost impossible," despite the evidence becoming insurmountable for those looking.

Perhaps boxing was closing ranks as Dr. Edith Summerskill, Labour MP in the United Kingdom, was arguing for the sport to be abolished. In fact, Summerskill and British promoter Jack Solomons were involved in a public war about the sport's future. Solomons, who had worked with hundreds of fighters and dominated the UK landscape in the 1950s and '60s, insisted he had not seen one case of punch-drunkenness and therefore argued in favor of the sport. Summerskill felt so strongly about the subject that she wrote a book arguing against the sport called *The Ignoble Art*. She also felt so vehemently about Solomons that she dedicated a chapter to him entitled "My Debate with Jack Solomons." The two came head-to-head to "discuss" the matter in 1953. With each side given twenty minutes to explain their beliefs, Summerskill brought a skull to articulate her points, while Solomons brought world light-heavyweight champion Freddie Mills. Summerskill went with the science, looking at anatomy and the structure of the brain as she exhausted her time, whereas Solomons spoke for only a few minutes. He argued that fighters who had made it had been able to set themselves up after boxing, buying bars, earning well, and one even marrying a rich woman. "What's wrong with the business if they can do that?" Solomons asked quizzically.

Fight journalist Peter Wilson also spoke for less than twenty minutes, as did Mills, who argued flimsily that boxing was a great sport because he was attending in an expensive suit, made by a top tailor, and he had a nice house and garden. He apparently received rapturous applause when he asked the lawyers in attendance whether they thought he was punch-drunk.

For fight historian Silver, Summerskill is something of a heroine. Silver had suffered migraines after that sparring session in his teens and subsequently read her work. "It's really obvious she hated the sport but it had absolutely no effect," Silver said. "You can't focus on the deaths in boxing. The deaths are awful, but the thing is to focus on those fighters who suffer the damage who don't die in the ring but whose lives are so diminished and whose intellectual capacity is affected because of the sport. If you go through *The Ring Record Book* and go down A through Z, I would say 80 percent of every fighter who has boxed beyond a certain point has some sort of brain damage, some worse than others."

But yet Solomons, the British Boxing Board of Control, and Freddie Mills were not alone in giving boxing a clean bill of health. Ira A. McCown, medical director of the New York State Athletic Commission and a qualified surgeon, still had not been sold on the idea that boxing was causing health issues in boxers. McCown wrote of punch-drunk syndrome,

"Acute cerebral trauma and its sequalae, chronic traumatic encephalopathy, have long been considered the most frequent serious complications of boxing. The so-called punch-drunk syndrome described by Martland over thirty years ago has become symbolic of brain injury. It has never been proved to be a neurological syndrome peculiar to boxers and produced by boxing. It has, unfortunately, become a slick medical cliché with which to label any boxer whose performance and behavior in or out of the ring is unsatisfactory or abnormal."

McCown's paper flew in the face of other medical experts in a flat-out denial of punch-drunk syndrome. Along with a team of researchers, he looked at EEG scans and physically examined fighters. McCown's research was astonishing. "During the past seven years, over 11,000 boxers have been examined and licensed in New York State. Twenty old, retired boxers were examined, and 148 boxers out of the total number were retired or refused a license because of medical disability," McCown continued. "Not one of the boxers examined revealed a typical punch-drunk syndrome. We have no evidence at hand to prove that such a syndrome exists in boxers."

McCown contended that safety measures including the ring canvas having more padding, heavier gloves, properly fitted mouthpieces, a portable resuscitator at ringside, and mandatory thirty-day suspensions for fighters who were stopped or knocked out had made the game safer. Then, in his conclusion, he hammered home his point with a finishing right hand: "No clinical or laboratory evidence was found which would substantiate the so-called punch-drunk syndrome that has so often been erroneously identified with boxers."

Whether McCown's role at the New York State Athletic Commission played a part in his findings is not known, but there were plenty who disagreed. Critchley would later counter that his own neurological experiences had revealed more than a hundred neurological cases. "Many of these—perhaps even the majority—should be looked upon as examples of punch-drunkenness, either early or well established," he said.

* * *

In May 1956, Johnny Bratton—a former welterweight champion who had boxed the likes of Kid Gavilan, Johnny Saxton, Ralph "Tiger" Jones, Holly Mims, and many other top-drawer stars—was working his way through several Illinois state hospitals. An old man at thirty, he stayed at the Manteno State Hospital, a psychiatric hospital, for eight years and then moved in with his mother. He was homeless for a while, slept in his car, and again was in and out of institutions. His torture continued for decades. He ran errands for change and wound up sleeping in the lobby of a seedy Chicago hotel. He lived in the past and off his old memories. He died in a nursing home in 1993. Decades had been lost to the punches he had taken. He was sixty-five.

Elsewhere, his former opponent Saxton lived into old age but did so in an impaired manner. First, he went off the rails. Having squandered a quarter of a million dollars in his career earnings, he was charged in 1959 with burglary, which got him a measly $5.20. He was destitute and owed the government about $20,000 in back taxes. The depth of Saxton's fall was revealed in court. He had been a brilliant fighter but he fought for the Mob and won and lost contests on their say-so.

"Johnny, where did your money go?" asked the judge.

Quietly slurring, Saxton replied, "I didn't get much of it."

"Why did you give up fighting?"

"They didn't need me no more."

Another man who could see what the business was like at the time was Paul Pender, a middleweight from Brookline, Massachusetts. He openly spoke up against the Mob but soon was forced to change his tune. "Boxing is rotten clear through, infested by gangsters and thieves," he said.

Pender had suffered with brittle hands and while medical bosses had been calling for a ban on the sport because fighters had been injured and killed in the ring, Pender thought the game should be abolished because of the criminals who ran it. In fact, there were as many calls to can the sport based on corruption as there were based on medical grounds.

"Why should boxing as it is conducted today be allowed to exist? So many fighters have been and are manipulated by despicable gangsters like Frankie Carbo. The public has lost all confidence in the sport," Pender vented.

It was, after all, in June 1960 when Jake LaMotta was forced to admit he had taken a dive in his fight with Billy Fox to get a middleweight title shot. But when Pender, a former Marine, was called on to explain his comments to the Massachusetts Boxing Commission, he said that his quotes had been taken out of context, that his comments had been "misconstrued," and that he had gotten his information from the newspapers—there was no wrongdoing in Massachusetts. Everyone knew that was not the case.

The threat of being frozen out of the title picture or being whisked away for a "gangland ride" and never returning was too real.

New York's "Irish" Jimmy Flood was a middleweight contender whose career overlapped Pender's in the 1950s. His wife, Dorothy, claimed he had suffered "brain damage" from his career after he was arrested on a wife-beating charge, and he was sent to Bellevue Hospital for psychological observation. Decades after Ad Wolgast, Terry McGovern, and Joe Grim had been kept in asylums, it was happening again. The diagnosis might no longer be punch-drunk, but the symptoms were the same.

Alas, poor Freddie Mills, the Bournemouth light heavyweight who'd fought in the corner of promoter Jack Solomons, wound up as one of boxing's most mysterious cases. He had competed over and over in the old boxing booths, sometimes against opponents who massively outweighed him and sometimes five or six times a day. He had 101 pro fights, boxing for money for fifteen years, and competing in more than 700 rounds. He died in 1965 of a gunshot wound to the head. It's a death that remains unsolved. Some said he owed large sums of money to London gangsters; others said he committed suicide. Chris Evans, who later wrote *Fearless Freddie: The Life and Times of Freddie Mills*, reckoned he had been suffering from chronic traumatic encephalopathy.

A year later, another British boxing great, middleweight Randolph Turpin took his own life. Bankrupt, owing back taxes, and the patient of a doctor who'd declared him punch-drunk, he'd become paranoid and was found with two gunshot wounds, one that had penetrated his skull but didn't make it to his brain, the other through his heart. His seventeen-month-old daughter Carmen was also discovered with two bullet wounds but made a full recovery.

"Randy Turpin and Freddie Mills," considered boxing historian Silver. "You have those guys who committed suicide. I wish their brains had been studied . . . did the brain damage contribute to Randy Turpin's suicide? The man was penniless. His life had fallen apart. I'm sure the brain damage was there, but I guarantee you could have carried on a conversation with Randy Turpin just before he committed suicide. Freddie Mills no doubt suffered brain damage, no question, and it might have been depression, but I'm sure it was compounded by [the fact that] these guys

[were] out of the limelight and [had] turned to drink and so on, but there's no question they suffered brain damage."

✱ ✱ ✱

Of course, it wasn't all boxers who were affected. Silver wondered why brawlers like Carmen Basilio, Jake LaMotta, Tony DeMarco, and Joe Miceli were comparatively unscathed and he had a layperson's theory: "I found out all of these guys were converted southpaws," he said. "A good friend of mine named Mike Capriano Jr., who is one of the greatest boxing minds I've ever met, he was the son of the trainer who discovered LaMotta and he himself had been an amateur boxer. He became a lawyer and he managed boxers. We were talking about this and he said they were all converted southpaws—in other words they were left-handed, and in those days nobody would fight a lefty so they turned them around, like they did in public school. Kids who were left-handed they made write with [their] right hand. So these guys, at a young age who were sixteen, seventeen, eighteen, the trainers were re-augmenting their brains to do things that didn't come natural to them, so instead of leading with their left hand they switched around to lead with their right. Now what did this do? By changing their whole orientation from left-handed to be right-handed, what does that do to the brain? It creates new neural connections and this to us was an explanation for this. Not that they didn't have brain trauma, but since they had these other connections that most people don't have . . . they had a reserve to fall back on when their sixties and early seventies came around. If they had [taken] that same damage and didn't have that same reserve to fall back on [that was] created by the neural pathways, they would have been mumbling by the time they were in their sixties or whatever."

Silver's assertions might sound like a shot in the dark, but in Ernst Jokl's *The Medical Aspect of Boxing*, there was a possible link buried under decades of research. Jokl had worked with Fritz Rolauf, a former German featherweight champion from Berlin, who contended that boxing helped develop the functioning capacity of the brain when arguing the case for the sport. "He tries to explain his theory," Jokl wrote, "by saying that training of the left arm leads to stimulation of a portion of the brain which is otherwise not used. He also alleges that many schoolteachers have told him that class performances of their pupils have become better, that their attention, their keenness, and their industry have improved after they had taken up boxing, 'especially after they had practiced their left arms.'"

But, of course, DeMarco, Miceli, LaMotta, and Basilio were exceptions, not the rule.

And the Murderers' Row struggled during and after boxing. Holman Williams died in a fire in 1967. Eddie Booker, who had been forced to retire with an eye injury, died in 1975 when his heart stopped. Aaron Wade died in 1985 at the age of sixty-eight. He had been getting ready for his own retirement party, having left his job at the Gallo Wine warehouse. Jack Chase, who had suffered with alcoholism, died in 1972. He had diabetes and pancreatitis. Bert Lytell died in a hospital in 1990. Charley Burley was, for many, the best on that unfortunate row. He had slowed to the point of speaking in a whisper and died in 1992 having made it to seventy-five. Lloyd Marshall developed Alzheimer's and Cocoa Kid had dementia pugilistica, dying alone in a Veterans Administration Hospital in Chicago on December 27, 1966. A veteran of 249 fights, he was only fifty-two.

* * *

Earlier in 1966, Professor Henry Miller from the Department of Neurology at the Royal Victoria Infirmary in Newcastle upon Tyne in England wrote a paper entitled "Mental After-effects of Head Injury." Miller was investigating compensation claims and trying to identify the legitimacy of those medical-legal cases, be it from workplace accidents, road traffic incidents, or crashes involving motorcyclists. He was analyzing behavior in claimants to determine whether they warranted payouts. Miller was a cynical man, but in conclusion, he wrote that, "It seems on the other hand that this syndrome, graphically described as 'punch-drunk,' is an authentic result of repeated cerebral injury."

Miller ran through researchers C. Mawdsley and F. R. Ferguson's list of symptoms from 1963 and agreed with their analysis: poor speech, tremors, unsteadiness, and depression.

No, Miller did not think repeated injuries to the brain provided anyone with a "slick medical cliché." He thought it was altogether more serious than that. He wrote that such repeated injuries to the brain gave you chronic traumatic encephalopathy, which would later become known around the world, in medical journals and popular culture, as CTE.

4
The Collector

UNTOLD STORIES FROM
THE BRAIN

As the 1970s roared around and Joe Frazier and Muhammad Ali borrowed against their future well-being to dig oh-so-deep in the "Fight of the Century" in 1971—the one in which Ali scraped himself off the canvas from a skull-crushing left hook to see out the tumultuous fifteen rounds only to lose on the scorecards—neurologists were starting to take a closer look at what was going on inside a fighter's head. They weren't exploring what made fighters tick, nor what separated the champions from contenders and journeymen, but what was happening to the brain after it had been subjected to a career of abuse.

A couple of years before that historic Madison Square Garden showdown, Anthony Herber Roberts published a book called *Brain Damage in Boxers: A Study of the Prevalence of Traumatic Encephalopathy Among Ex-Professional Boxers.* He investigated the long-term health and well-being of 224 professional prizefighters (out of a pool of 16,781 active boxers) who had been registered with the British Boxing Board of

Control between 1929 and 1955. The subjects were examined clinically and through EEG scans.

Roberts's work was the result of another epic tussle, but one outside the ropes, when in 1962 the House of Lords in Britain discussed the legality of boxing. The ironically named neurologist Walter Russell Brain, prompted by Dr. Edith Summerskill, asked lawmakers to consider the sport's future and Roberts was tasked with examining what happened to fighters and their health after the final bell had tolled. London's Royal College of Physicians had also urged Roberts to complete the study.

Roberts was a terrific researcher whose work painted a vivid picture. His 132-page magnum opus delved into the health and backgrounds of prizefighters and he argued that "there is a danger of chronic brain damage occurring in boxers as a result of their careers." Roberts found that of thirty-seven cases, 17 percent had dementia pugilistica and thirteen of the boxers were permanently disabled.

Roberts attempted to establish sequences and patterns by assessing how many fights a boxer had taken part in, over how many years, how much sparring a fighter had done, what skills the boxer had, how old he was when he started and retired, and how many times he had been knocked out. Half of Roberts's group over the age of fifty who had fought for at least a decade were damaged, as were around half of those who boxed more than 150 times. The longer the career, the more likely the harm. Roberts could see lesions on the brain that he thought might form a chronic, clinical syndrome. "Chronic" meant progressive, that there might not be signs at first but that there would be deterioration over time.

Given that Harrison Martland's "Punch Drunk" paper had been written almost fifty years earlier, it was a damning indictment of the lack of cohesiveness between those in boxing and those in the medical profession that, at a similar time Roberts went about his work, neuropathologist John Arthur Nicholas Corsellis and his colleagues wrote, "It is not easy to establish a pattern of damage or of degeneration in such limited material and most of the trenchant views that are expressed about the vulnerability, as well as the immunity, of the brain in boxing are still based more on supposition than on fact."

There had just not been enough research yet. Despite the fighters and their afflictions, there was nothing saying that boxing was causing any of it, just that it was happening to boxers. Despite the depth of his study, Roberts was still missing something. There was a lot of "boxing could . . ." and "boxing might . . ." but there was no evidence that boxing *did* anything. The evidence was circumstantial and could still be put down to coincidence.

But Corsellis had been collecting brains since 1951 and had accumulated several that had belonged to former fighters. His library of untold secrets of trauma was somewhat morbidly called the "Corsellis Collection," and it was housed at the Department of Neurology at the Institute of Psychiatry at Runwell Hospital in Wickford, Essex. Corsellis meticulously combed through the Roberts report and looked at the brains of fifteen prizefighters who had boxed as youngsters, twelve of whom had turned professional, with eight going on to win regional, national, or even world honors. They had died between the ages of fifty-seven and ninety-one and had all passed away from natural causes. But there was nothing natural about Corsellis's approach. Along with a team of researchers—C. J. Bruton and Dorothy Freeman-Browne—he set about matching patterns in the brains with the fighters' behavior. They interviewed those who had known the boxers well—family, friends, wives, girlfriends, trainers, children, social workers, and doctors—as they tried to detect personality traits while matching them to the pathology in the brain.

All fifteen fighters had suffered from punch-drunk syndrome, or dementia pugilistica, and the autopsies showed severe irregularities and cerebral atrophy in fourteen of the fifteen. In time, those changes would be seen as key components of dementia pugilistica and Corsellis, owner of what would become the largest brain bank in Europe before it closed in 2010, had actually discovered punch-drunk syndrome in fighters.

Among those changes in the impaired brains, the septum—a vertical wall that separates the left and right side of the brain—was torn, and in some cases next to nothing remained. Punches had caused the separation of the septum pellucidum by the third ventricle. Based on 142 studies, in non-boxers, the space in the separation averaged 1.6 mm (0.06 inches), but in fighters, the gap was 5.17 mm (0.20 inches). Corsellis believed the structural differences could have resulted in changes to a fighter's emotions, whether he suffered from rage and depression, which as it turned out many athletes in his study had. He also said the gap, which would be attributed to punches, was "the rule rather than the exception."

Corsellis speculated how the exposure to different types of punches—rotational and accelerative forces—might damage the brain.

One of the two world champions whose brains Corsellis studied had been a bright child at school, started boxing at eleven, was married, popular, and became a world champion. His change in circumstances was shocking. His marriage disintegrated, and bar the occasional "embarrassing visit," he drifted from his family, had violent tendencies, could not hold a job, and, at age sixty-three, "was found lying neglected and louse-ridden in the boiler house of a hotel." While in the hospital, he slurred his words, was unsteady on his feet, and died several months later.

The second world champion had boxed from boyhood, fought a few times a day in the old "blood tubs," and went on to win a world title. In total, he had an estimated seven hundred fights, retiring in his early thirties. By then, his family said, he was "a little old man . . . playing the part of an animated punching bag." By fifty he staggered when he walked, had slurred speech, and "you'd think he was always drunk but he never touched a drop." Then his memory deserted him. At sixty-seven he became so confused and disorientated it was like looking after a child. He remembered only sections of his boxing career and "he often wanted to be cuddled and reassured . . . he would sulk when left alone and smile happily when approached." He could not stand on one leg without falling over, suffered with tremors, and was diagnosed with punch-drunk syndrome. He somehow made it to age seventy-seven, demented and incontinent before dying in a psychiatric hospital.

The other cases were no less tragic. One fighter began to get muddled at the age of thirty-six, by which time he would occasionally fall over or experience paranoia; and then, by age fifty, he had slurred speech and tremors. His widow told researchers how he got worse, endured moments of fury and then complete calm, and died at age sixty-three.

Case after case painted a similar picture, and after each background presentation, Corsellis recorded the appearance of the fighter's brain and histological (tissue structure) findings, while analyzing the brain stem (the rear of the brain that links it to the spinal cord) and the cerebellum (the part that receives information from the sensory systems, including the spinal cord and other parts of the brain). In the back of the cerebellum, where motor movements are controlled, Corsellis found scarring in ten of the fifteen fighters, and punches had seemingly caused the cerebellum to push down on the foramen magnum, which produced scarring and affected a boxer's speech, balance, and motor movements.

The substantia nigra, a structure contained deep within the brain that when damaged has been linked with Parkinson's, had been annihilated so clearly in several fighters' brains that Corsellis didn't even need a microscope to see it. Indeed, four of the fighters had been hospitalized and diagnosed with Parkinson's.

In addition, Corsellis found traces of tangles of protein spread around the hippocampus and other sections of the brain, the same tangles found in Alzheimer's sufferers. There was further damage to the limbic system, the headquarters involving memory and learning. The increase in neurofibrillary tangles (clumps of toxic protein) were specifically found in the medial temporal lobe. Such tangles had been seen in the elderly population, linked to senile plaques, but the tangles were seen in fourteen of fifteen fighters. However, nine of them had not one senile plaque, so Corsellis determined that the tangles had appeared because of head trauma and not senility.

Some boxers in the case studies also suffered from severe depression. At least one admitted to attempting suicide. Several saw out their last days in psychiatric units, still without anyone knowing what had actually happened to them and their brains and why. There was a standout who died at age ninety-one and who was "a remarkably well-preserved old man" and two who did not become symptomatic at all. But other than that, there was a trail of splintered relationships and deteriorating health—physical and mental—with some or all of the trademark physical signs of punch-drunkenness.

Corsellis's discoveries were huge. His paper was called "Aftermath of Boxing" and was published in *Psychological Medicine* in 1973. "There is still a danger that, at an unpredictable moment and for an unknown reason, one or more blows will leave their mark," he wrote. "The destruction of cerebral tissue will have then begun, and although this will usually be slight enough in the early stage to be undetectable, it may build up, if the boxing continues, until it becomes clinically evident. At this point, however, it could already be too late."

Unlike the neurologists who came before him, Corsellis believed that the fighters who were the most at risk were the better, more successful ones. They had the longest careers, fought the best opponents, and took more shots to the head.

The argument was echoed years later by former *Boxing News* editor Claude Abrams, who had become uneasy watching the sport, having witnessed the damage to so many fighters during his two decades at ringside. He thought it was a misconception that those likely to suffer were boxers who were involved in mismatches or lesser-skilled fighters. "From my experience, the opposite is true," said Abrams. "The lasting damage tends to come from long fights, where boxers take repeated punches. Most vulnerable are the brave, the tough, the durable, and those with the greatest will. They are often the best. When you match the best against the best, the fight is equal. There is no give. The duration of these matches is usually longer and the quality and accuracy of punches greater. The stakes and desire to win are higher. Consequently, these boxers push themselves to the limit."

✳ ✳ ✳

Thus it was becoming an outdated belief that only journeymen, sparring partners, or fighters with losing records would suffer. All-time greats were in trouble, too—the likes of Joe Louis, Henry Armstrong, and Sugar Ray Robinson.

And then there was the legendary "Cincinnati Cobra," Ezzard Charles. Charles was one of the best light heavyweights in history and even managed to move up in weight to capture the world heavyweight title, which he held between 1949 and 1951. In 1954, deeply underappreciated and a faded force at that, he lost to Rocky Marciano, who would refer to Charles as "the bravest man I ever fought."

This is a sport in which bravery can be measured by the amount of punishment one can withstand.

Charles boxed another twenty-three times, losing often. He wound up with ninety-five wins against twenty-five defeats and a draw. He was stopped seven times. His last contest was in September 1959 when he was thirty-eight, almost twenty years after turning professional. Until he got his big break, he had worked his way up and down Murderers' Row.

But in 1973, just fourteen years after calling it a day, Charles appeared in a nationwide commercial on U.S. television. Interspersed with clips of him landing bombs against rival Jersey Joe Walcott, Charles was in a boxing ring. The black-and-white arena was empty. It was silent as the camera, from the bleachers, panned in on him. He sat in a wheel-chair. The ring ropes were loose, the ringside seats were vacant. He was tipping over to his left in the chair and a narrator said that in 1968 Charles had contracted ALS, a neuromuscular disease that was related to organs or tissues wasting. "It left him helpless as a baby," the audience was told.

At the end of the commercial, the camera moved in closer still, showing the ex-fighter's expressionless eyes, and the narrator concluded: "Ezzard Charles is still fighting, but this time it's for his life. Help Ezzard Charles and thousands like him in their fight against neuromuscular diseases. Give what you can, but give." A caption then appeared on screen that read, "Help our fight. Muscular Dystrophy Association of America."

Charles had been a busy professional. Even after winning the title he fought often and then, when he lost it, he was like a gambler playing bad hands night after night trying to get it all back using reduced speed, power, and reflexes—meanwhile his mileage increased. His decline followed a familiar pattern that included refusal, denial, rejection, and then grim acceptance.

As Charles hit his early thirties, writers began telling him he was near the end through the questions they posed. (Once the writers ask a fighter how much longer is left, it shows that they see the finish line even if the fighter himself can't.) Charles was then floored, beaten, and stopped by the average Chicago heavyweight Johnny Holman, who could never have stood with Charles at his best. "The incentive's still the same as it was ten years ago," Charles told one reporter. "I'm still trying to do the same things. To build up to a title shot. Keep fighting to get into position for the championship. Of course, they pay you for boxing." But by that point they were paying for Charles's name as much as the fight.

When he eked by Paul Andrews on a split decision, Charles said, "Fighting is my business. I don't have another job. Besides, how can you turn down the money?"

He was running out of that and things were only going to get worse.

At thirty-four, Charles noticed a problem with his left ankle but kept it to himself. He was, by now, losing more than he was winning and in nothing like championship class. "I plan to go right on fighting until I detect that I have slowed up and have little to offer," he explained, not realizing that time had come.

One writer asked whether he would be able to see it happening. Perhaps the question was rhetorical. "Well, sometimes the athlete finds out about his slipping after spectators have noted it. But I am sure that I will be the first to know if I've begun to slide down the toboggan. The champion who outlasts his welcome is a sucker," said the depleted Charles.

He retired, under pressure from his wife, Gladys, but returned—as they do. She had pleaded with him to quit while he still had his health, but it was all he knew. He was short of cash and boxing was in him; it had manifested itself deep in his soul as it does with almost every fighter who feels a surge of excitement on the run-up to fight night that peaks with an adrenaline-soaked evening under the lights, in the ring. How do you replace that? Charles couldn't.

"I suppose all this would surprise a lot of people, but gosh, boxing was always my life," he said, explaining his return. "It was everything. I really miss all the cheers, and, yes, the jeers of my fighting days. It's a world all of its own. I have a fine job with a juvenile-detention home here. But it doesn't fill my needs. That's all."

More beatings came his way.

The ankle was becoming less responsive and he was battered into a severe loss by Texan Donnie Fleeman. Charles was suspended in the Lone Star state because of his dwindling fighting abilities and officials hoped other boxing commissions would follow suit.

But he was allowed to fight in Boise and, having made almost $250,000 against Rocky Marciano years earlier, Charles now earned just $200 for a fight in a high school gym. At thirty-eight, and after losing to Alvin Green, he said he would box for another three or four years. It was getting grim. "It's an easy way to make a living," he reckoned.

He did signings, opened bars, toyed with the idea of becoming a wrestler, made bad business decisions, and lost steady jobs. By 1965 his wife noticed that Charles was walking differently. "He'd be climbing stairs on his way from the office and there would be this sort of wobble in his walk," she said. "A sort of stumbling motion, like he was drunk or something. . . . He began to look like a drunk—not a bad drunk, more like a light drunk, one who has got a high."

Concerned, he went to the hospital to get checked over and was diagnosed with ALS, more commonly known as Lou Gehrig's disease. He and his wife didn't think it was boxing related, but ALS was a degeneration of the body that would cause it to break down in sections. The ankle would go into the leg. The muscles would get tight and then fail because they weren't being used. "First he would lose his ability to walk," wrote Charles's biographer William Detloff. "Soon he wouldn't be able to use his arms or shoulders. He would lose bladder and bowel control. Eventually he'd be unable to speak, and after that he wouldn't be able to swallow. Inevitably he would stop breathing too and then he would die by asphyxiation, probably within five years."

As Charles's condition worsened, a benefit night was held in his honor. By that point he was spending most of his waking hours in a wheelchair, but the one-thousand-strong audience celebrated his achievements. Joe Louis, Rocky Marciano, Muhammad Ali, Henry Armstrong, Joe Walcott, and Archie Moore were all there. Charles was called up to say a few words. He couldn't manage much but he wheeled his way to the center of the stage and was helped gingerly to his feet by Louis and Walcott. He used the podium to steady himself and murmured his appreciation, "This is the nicest thing that ever happened to me."

It was his last public appearance. Weeks and months went by, Gladys was by his side all the way.

In 1972, Charles had been confined to a wheelchair for six years and looking after him was all Gladys could do. She took him to the toilet, fed him, and tried to understand when he spoke until they had to work out their own language, a cross between the alphabet and blinking. She would do the letters and he would do the blinking. He was still only fifty-one. In 1973 he filmed the commercial for the Muscular Dystrophy Association of America and, as he deteriorated, Gladys was unable to look after him anymore. She put him into a VA hospital in 1974 and he spent two years in room B804 at the VA West Side Hospital in Chicago on Damen Avenue with Gladys a regular, loving visitor. He died on May 28, 1975, aged fifty-three, almost twenty years after he first noticed a problem with his ankle.

While there were thousands suffering from ALS across the United States, no one had linked it to boxing or multiple traumatic brain injuries. It wasn't until the early 2000s that correlations were made between football players and ALS. The percentage of former professionals suffering with the condition was far higher than it statistically should have been.

The disease had been named after the baseball superstar Lou Gehrig, who died from it in 1941 at the age of thirty-seven. Yet the illness and how people got it remained a mystery. There were no links between Gehrig and head injuries until 2010 when an HBO documentary team found images of Gehrig being aided from the field after being knocked out from a ball to the head and another of him unconscious from a collision on the field. In total he had suffered at least six serious head injuries. And for Gehrig, it perhaps wasn't just the blows to the head that contributed to his illness; it was also the failure to treat his injuries properly. There was no rest for the cult figure who was known as "Iron Horse" for his famous "streak," playing 2,130 consecutive games, including six games that came immediately after the six head injuries. It's possible that the "streak" he became so famous for played a significant role in his health collapsing and his death, just a couple of years after he'd been forced to retire.

✳ ✳ ✳

Meanwhile, one wondered if a young Minnesota heavyweight called Scott LeDoux ever saw the Ezzard Charles commercial; he turned professional in 1974, just a year after its release. LeDoux boxed for less than a decade, had fifty bouts, but died at sixty-two.

Ironically, he had been close with Wally Hilgenberg, an ALS sufferer who played as a linebacker for the Minnesota Vikings. LeDoux witnessed Hilgenberg's disintegration and then found out it was about to take hold of him. "I went to visit Wally and he was unable to communicate with us," said LeDoux, who faced eleven world champions from Muhammad Ali to George Foreman and Ken Norton to Michael Spinks, joking that boxing was a Christian sport—much better to give than receive. "It was pretty scary for me," LeDoux said.

After his boxing career, LeDoux became involved in the politics in Minnesota but was diagnosed with ALS in 2008. In 2010 he resigned from his role as Anoka county commissioner, citing his ailing health, and he went to a county board meeting to make the announcement. "He stood up from his wheelchair for the Pledge of Allegiance," county chairman Dennis Berg recalled. "That was a real struggle for him. But it was something he found the courage to do."

ALS sufferers experience degeneration of nerve cells in their central nervous system. Only around 20 percent of sufferers live five years or more after developing ALS and it was shutting the popular Minnesotan down.

"It's unbelievable that I admitted it—ALS is taking my life," he said in a 2010 interview. He believed boxing had been a physical fight while ALS was a mental battle. "It's emotional because you're going to die," he said. "I've got three grandsons and I want to be around for them."

LeDoux's wife looked after him 24/7. He would still joke occasionally because, he said, "I want to laugh, I don't want to cry." And for a while he could get around using Hilgenberg's old walker after his friend passed away. LeDoux knew his days were numbered and he signed legal documents that said, "When I can't breathe anymore, it's going to be done."

He died in 2011.

During an autopsy, doctors checked Hilgenberg's brain and spinal cord. He always suspected his damage may have been from football but he never knew. They found toxic proteins that form after head trauma and poison the brain. The toxins had also made their way into Hilgenberg's spinal column and poisoned his nervous system. Soon after, similar discoveries were made in another football player and a boxer whose family did not want him identified.

* * *

Several decades after Charles passed away, a Boston University study found possible links between ALS and CTE in contact sportsmen and women after families of twelve athletes made tissue donations to the VA-BU-CLF Brain Bank at the Bedford, Massachusetts, VA Medical Center.

Three years after LeDoux passed away, the great former light-heavyweight champion Matthew Saad Muhammad died, also from ALS. He had fought on way too long, had a horrible in-ring decline where he traveled the world trying to get a license to fight in his worn-out state, and often getting one as local commissions tried to cash in on his name. ALS had a grip on him for years. He also exhibited other physical symptoms of a long career: short-term memory loss, aggression, imbalanced gait, slurred speech. He was fifty-nine when he died. His fortunes from a series of highlight-reel WBC light-heavyweight title defenses—some of the greatest ring wars of all time—had been squandered long ago. He lived in a homeless shelter for a while, recalled seeing only flashing lights and shadows from his historic battles against fighters like Marvin Johnson and Yaqui Lopez, and when he finally died, penniless, he was buried in an unmarked grave. Boxing historian John DiSanto, who helps preserve Philadelphia's fight heritage, raised money from fans online to pay for a headstone.

But back when Charles was used as a tragic poster boy for a national campaign, scientists were not looking at ALS in relation to boxing. They had been trying to establish what punch-drunk syndrome was, what dementia pugilistica was, and what CTE was. Charles just had an illness anyone could have gotten. That was the consensus.

But Corsellis and his collection of brains began to solve the mysteries that had been posed decades earlier.

5
Poster Boys

A LABEL NOBODY WANTS

As the 1960s neared an end, Muhammad Ali was starting over. His claim that he had no quarrel with the Vietcong had cost him three years, and by 1970 he was free to fight again.

Ali was a different boxer following his enforced sabbatical. In his first incarnation, he was a flighty mover; on his return, he'd become a gritty but somehow still-elegant slugger.

He was matched tough for his comeback, paired with California hardman Jerry Quarry. Ali was 29-0 and considered ring rusty. Quarry was an experienced 37-4-4. They met in Atlanta, and by the end of the third round, Ali had disproved notions of decay and his hand was raised. Quarry was bleeding heavily from a cut over his left eye, which had needed fifteen stitches to close.

Quarry had never been the most elusive boxer. "There's no quit in a Quarry" was the family's fighting mantra, instilled into three boxing siblings by their father, Jack. But Ali had changed, and as the years of his comeback wore on, he would depend upon his chin rather than his footwork, his determination rather than his ambition, and his experience rather than his youth.

Yes, he could turn back the clock and dominate on his terms against lesser men, but often—as he grew older—he would lure heavy hitters in using his rope-a-dope tactics, absorb an opponent's hardest shots, ideally on the arms and gloves (though not exclusively), and retaliate after he had weathered the storm. The most famous case came in Zaire in 1974 when the feared and favored George Foreman smashed away repeatedly at the smaller man before wilting in the historic African night in round eight.

But through these fights, Ali's fight doctor had noticed cumulative issues. Dr. Ferdie Pacheco could see warning signs in training when Ali did the same thing over and over in the gym. He would take his back to the ropes, lift his arms, tuck his chin in, and start trying to ride everything that came his way. It was a painful way to make a living, and it made his sparring sessions at Deer Lake in Pennsylvania ridiculously exciting as Ali staved off the ferocious attacks from men who were hired to knock lumps out of him.

Ali slowed and slowed. In 1978, he survived fifteen rounds with the heaviest puncher in the division's history, when Earnie Shavers hit Ali so hard that Ali said "it shook my kinfolk in Africa." Ali won that one but then lost to former Olympic champion, seven-fight professional novice Leon Spinks in an upset, before correcting that wrong in another bruising encounter seven months later.

Then there were two hard, heartbreaking losses: a whitewash ten-round stoppage defeat to former sparring partner Larry Holmes and a farce in the Bahamas when Ali was allowed—crazily—to go ten more rounds with a young Trevor Berbick.

Quarry was also on the decline, blitzed in five by Joe Frazier and Ken Norton. He retired in November 1983, almost two years after Berbick had brutalized the remnants of Ali.

But Ali and Quarry were in trouble.

Their paths had crossed again in 1972, with Ali winning the rematch in seven in Las Vegas, but a decade later they were in the same fight.

Following the fatal bout between Ray Mancini and the tragic Duk Koo Kim, *Sports Illustrated* assigned Robert H. Boyle to write about brain damage in boxers.

By that point in 1983, it could and should have been different for Ali. He had fought when he had nothing left to prove, took paydays when his name would have always held value, and taken punches when he should have been making his mark in a new life after boxing. Ali was another addict captured by the big-fight extravagance, magnetized by the media, energized by the crowds—a host to the world, a showman who couldn't live without a show.

Years earlier, with the damage yet to truly set in, Ali was asked about his exit strategy. He said, "I don't want to be one of them old fighters with a hat nose [who] say 'duh duh duh' before a fight."

Things didn't work out the way he hoped. By the time he said those words, Ali was already deteriorating. While Boyle did reach Ali— who declined to be interviewed for the *Sports Illustrated* article—the forty-one-year-old Ali had conceded "it's possible" that he was slowing down because of an accumulation of punches. The writer noted that Ali "has been slurring his words and acting depressed of late." But Ali wouldn't take part in the neurological testing the publication wanted him to, claiming his results had been 'normal' in previous tests through 1980 and 1981, though 'normal' was up for debate, and the interpretation of the findings varied enormously.

Through the *Sports Illustrated* investigation, Boyle found that Ali had a cavum septum pellucidum, which can be seen on a CAT scan and is not wholly unusual for the man on the street, but something that is incredibly common in prizefighters. He also had an enlarged third ventricle. They got the information from a scan Ali had done before the last fight of his career, but the scan had come back "negative"—or normal.

According to the *Sports Illustrated* piece, "Most neuroradiologists aren't familiar with the scans of boxers. They don't know that the atrophy like that found on Ali's scan show up in 50 percent of boxers with more than 20 bouts—a percentage far higher than in the general population, and that, by other criteria, these same boxers often show evidence of brain impairment. The cavum abnormality is found four times as frequently in boxers as in non-boxers."

In addition to Quarry and Randall "Tex" Cobb, *Sports Illustrated* used bantamweight journeyman Mark Pacheco in their investigation. (Quarry, by the way, said he was hoping to come out of retirement.) Pacheco had his boxing license revoked after getting knocked out in May 1982. He was suspended from fighting in Oregon for forty-five days but crept in under the radar and fought in New York forty-three days later, where he was knocked out again.

Quarry and Cobb were sure they were fine. Enter Ira Casson, a New York neurologist at the Long Island Jewish Medical Center. He had completed a study in the *British Journal of Neurology, Neurosurgery and Psychiatry* using CT scans, a comparatively new way of looking at the brain via an improved form of X-ray. Looking at nine pros, Casson scanned and examined them shortly after they had been knocked out and a tenth fighter who had been stopped. Five of the fighters showed signs of brain damage. Three of the fighters who had become world champions showed signs of damage, a fourth came up clear on the scans but was muddled and his short-term memory was bad.

Casson explored the number of fights they'd had and determined that five who had more than twenty bouts were damaged, while of the five with fewer than a dozen fights only one scan came back with the cavum septum pellucidum. Casson also recognized that in many ways the better fighters were at risk: they stayed on their feet for longer, could withstand punches better, and while they were more durable in their primes, they would pay for it down the line.

But for Ali, the warning signs had been there. He was known for his stubbornness—it was part of what made him such an outstanding fighter—but he was also known to not like people who told him things he didn't want to hear, and that had happened in 1976. Upon his return to the sport, he'd defeated a roll call of future Hall of Famers, contenders and nonentities who came and went in equal measure: Floyd Patterson, George Chuvalo, Joe Frazier, Ron Lyle—and, of course, George Foreman and Ken Norton. He won almost everything, and then came the sad collapse with his prime years in the rearview mirror.

Ali started to take punches in 1954, as a twelve-year-old. His final fight was a timid loss to Berbick over ten rounds in December 1981. Ali traded his name for $1.1 million that night in the Bahamas. He had fought sixty-one pro fights in a little more than two decades.

But the silence was beginning to shackle him, and by 1996, at the opening ceremony of the Atlanta Olympic Games, the depth of Ali's decline shocked a worldwide audience as, hands violently shaking, he tried to light the Olympic flame.

Ali became one of the most recognizable faces of Parkinson's syndrome. He started to show neurological deficiencies in the early 1980s, while he was still fighting, and he degenerated in front of the world that idolized him. It is still not wholly accepted that Ali had CTE, it's just that his symptoms were similar and without autopsy results it will never be known.

In 2017, a study that tracked his public speaking from 1968 to 1981 found that while he was in his thirties, he started slurring his words, years before he was diagnosed with Parkinson's syndrome at the age of forty-two. Arizona State University speech scientists Visar Berisha and Julie Liss measured the rate of syllables Ali spoke at and monitored how it decreased per second between the ages of twenty-six and thirty-nine. They observed signs of deterioration as early as 1978, three years before his last contest and six years before his diagnosis.

Meanwhile, pre-Berbick, Ali's entourage was still extravagant, but the personnel was changing. Longtime doctor Pacheco was gone. He had wanted Ali to retire after his third fight with Frazier, saying he would no longer be around if he fought beyond Shavers in 1978. So Pacheco left.

Author Thomas Hauser got to know the man universally referred to as "The Greatest" as well as anyone. He wrote *Muhammad Ali: His Life and Times,* the award-winning authorized biography and definitive Ali book, spending a considerable amount of time with Ali and his wife, Lonnie.

"The legs are the first thing to go in a fighter," Pacheco told Hauser for his book. "And when Ali went into exile, he lost his legs. Before that he'd been so fast you couldn't catch him, so he'd never taken punches. He'd been knocked down by Henry Cooper and Sonny Banks, but the truth is he rarely got hit and he'd never taken a beating. In the gym, he'd work with Luis Rodriguez, who was the fastest welterweight in the world and Luis, who was like lightning, couldn't hit him. Then, after the layoff, Ali came back and his legs weren't like they'd been before. And when he lost his legs, he lost his first line of defense. That was when he discovered something which was both very good and very bad. Very bad in that it led to the physical damage he suffered later in his career, very good in that it eventually got him back the championship. He discovered he could take a punch."

Pacheco thought the incredible violence Ali shared with Frazier in 1975 in Manila was the beginning of the end and that the abuse Ali absorbed in sparring to the kidneys and to the brain in his second spell, post-exile, marked a downward turn in his health. It was after the Shavers fight when the matchmaker at Madison Square Garden, Teddy Brenner, threw the towel in on his business association with Ali. "Champ, why don't you announce your retirement?" Brenner began. "What for?" came the reply. "Because sooner or later some kid that couldn't carry your bucket is going to beat you. You're going to be beaten by guys that have no business being in the ring with you. It's just a matter of time. If you take a big piece of iron and put it down on the center of the floor and let a drop of water hit it every ten seconds, eventually you'll get a whole in the center of that piece of iron, and that's what's happening to you. You're getting hit. You're getting hurt. . . . You don't need this. Get out."

Ali's once colorful and vibrant features were dimming. Pacheco would confide in Hauser, "If this is what boxing does, then it shouldn't be a sport. But this is not what boxing does. This is what boxing does if you stay on too long. Age thirty is the cusp. Thirty-five is over the line. I don't care how good you are, after age thirty-five you're getting brain damage. If Ali had quit when he should have quit, he wouldn't be having these problems today. But he didn't, and now you see what happened. . . ."

Pacheco later recalled to a documentary crew how he saw the signs of Ali's physical decline, urging them to look at the deterioration from one fight to the next.

"And if you continue like this, you're going to have massive brain damage, which is going to lead to the other neurological disorders, either Parkinson's or mid-brain damage, which is exactly like Parkinson's," warned Pacheco.

For Brenner and Pacheco it was like watching a car heading off a cliff. They didn't want to be the rubberneckers watching a tragedy unfold, complicit with aiding and abetting a decline they predicted. Ali's trainer Angelo Dundee was often criticized for being complicit with his fighter boxing on, but he contended he wanted to be the one in control in the corner and that he would be the one looking after him, not turning his back on him.

After the Shavers fight, Pacheco broke rank and sent Ali's post-fight medical report to Ali's wife, to Dundee, and to manager Herbert Muhammad, expressing his concerns, but he didn't hear back from any of them.

"Instead of filtering out blood and turning it into urine," Pacheco told Hauser, "pure blood was going through. That was bad news for the kidneys; and since everything in the body is interconnected, we were talking about the disintegration of Ali's health."

Years later, Pacheco lamented to *Sports Illustrated*, "He took some mammoth beatings. There were the fights with Frazier, Foreman, and Norton, to say nothing of all the sparring with Larry Holmes and Michael Dokes. Holmes and Dokes were not ordinary sparring partners. They're now heavyweight champions of the world. A moron could add up the picture of impending brain damage, and I urged him to quit because I didn't think it would be wonderful to have the most joyful, talented guy in the world stumbling around and mumbling to himself. But he was the one who wanted to stay on the stage. The only role he knew was being champion. I'd just as soon have been wrong."

By now the concerns were becoming more formal, too. Reporters put the Nevada State Athletic Commission under scrutiny. Could they not hear that Ali's voice was softer? Could they not see that his reflexes were going? Were they not aware that he'd been at this brutal business for nearly three decades?

In July 1980, Ali visited the Mayo Clinic in Rochester, Minnesota, for two days of renal and neurological testing having been told that he would not be licensed without it. Ali passed the physical test but that did not mean he was fit to fight. As Pacheco explained, in the mold of Harrison Martland decades earlier, "Most trainers can tell you better than any neurologist in the world when a fighter is shot."

Boxing people *know*.

"Sugar Ray Robinson could pass every exam in the world at age forty-four, but he wasn't Sugar Ray Robinson anymore," Pacheco told Hauser. "It doesn't change, whether it's Wilfred Benitez and Edwin Rosario, who were 'shot' by the time they reached their mid-twenties; Thomas Hearns, who's 'shot' at thirty; Ali, Joe Louis. Anybody in the gym can see it before the doctors can, because the doctors, good doctors, are judging these fighters by the standards of ordinary people and the demands of ordinary jobs and you can't do that because these are professional fighters."

A couple of reports were sent to Nevada, one stating that Ali's general medical health was okay but another, later accessed by Hauser with permission of Ali, played down concerns, putting most of his symptoms down to tiredness—even as he struggled to hop on one leg and touch his nose with his index finger. That doctor knew only of Ali being shaken on two occasions in his life: against Sonny Liston and Bob Foster. Of course, not knowing boxing, he couldn't press him on being hurt by Shavers, the battering he took from Foreman, and that's even before you get to the Frazier wars. Another red flag in that report was "tingling" in his hands and the neurologist said Ali had been slurring for ten to twelve years when it hadn't been that long.

According to experts, Ali was fit to fight—despite the slurring, tingling, and constant "tiredness." He was green-lighted to face the young, hungry Larry Holmes and although he suffered the beating of his life, it still wasn't over.

He had surrendered his license in Nevada after losing to Holmes in Las Vegas but did not want to go out like that. So a thirty-doctor team at New York University studied him, with Harry Demopoulos at the helm. Demopoulos claimed there was no evidence that Ali had sustained damage to any vital organs and continued to say, "If the slurring were due to permanent damage, it would be there all the time." It was blamed on travel or general fatigue.

Still, U.S. commissions wouldn't grant Ali consent to fight, so he wound up meeting Berbick in the more relaxed jurisdiction of Nassau in the Bahamas. It was a disaster. Ali's mother spoke of the dread she felt about it. Even before Holmes, Cassius Clay Sr. went on record with his worries. "I thought he wasn't walking good," said Ali's father. "I thought maybe his hip was bothering him. I wasn't sure of his speech, either, but the way I look at it, that boy has been fighting since he was twelve years old. A man can only stand so many licks to the head."

Major U.S. television channels refused to make offers for the contest, and several journalists who'd covered Ali's career boycotted the trip. Yet Ali remained resolute. "They say I'm washed up," he countered. "They say I'm too old. That I'm finished. That I can't talk no more. That I've got brain damage. That I have bad kidneys. That I'm broke. That I'm sad. Oooooh, man. I've got so many critics to whup. So many newspaper people who think I'm dead. So many boxing commissions. So many doctors. I'm gonna mess 'em all up by whupping Berbick and then becoming the first forty-year-old man to ever win the heavyweight title. Get ready for the shocker. I'm gonna mess up the world."

Even logistically, the "event" was chaos. The stadium opened two hours late because no one could find a key, they didn't have a ring bell so they used a cowbell instead, and there were only two pairs of gloves so they were cut off each fighter's fists from the undercard all the way through. But none of that was the story. The story was that Ali shouldn't have been fighting, yet here he was having found one of boxing's many loopholes.

By now he cut a pitiful figure. No one ever wanted to see him beaten or humiliated by a man who could not touch him in his prime, yet that's what happened—he was outpointed over ten rounds.

"I think I'm too old," Ali finally conceded, his stomach with a paunchy look and hair dye hiding the gray. "I was slow. I was weak. Nothing but Father Time. The things I wanted to do, I couldn't do. I was doing my best. I did good for a thirty-nine-year-old. I think I'm finished. I know it's the end. I'm not crazy. After Holmes, I had excuses. I was too light. Didn't breathe right. No excuses this time. I'm happy. I'm still pretty. I could have a black eye. Broken teeth. Split lips. I think I came out all right for an old man."

The signs started to get rapidly worse. Within a few years he had filmed interviews with the BBC that they could not use because his speech was too far gone. He was asked, then, whether he might be punch-drunk. "I have heard about people being punch-drunk, but I do not feel drunk," he replied, jokingly. "When you're as great as me, people always look for some type of downfall."

Then, of course, the long and gloomy deterioration set in, punctuated by appearances that may have educated people about Parkinson's but that ultimately made a generation feel sorry for one of the most magnificent physical specimens of all time. Ali, "The Louisville Lip," was all but muted. He tremored rigorously and his once flashing footwork became increasingly sterile. The Ali shuffle simply became a shuffle.

It had been in 1984 when Ali realized he couldn't hide the truth from himself any longer. Writer George Plimpton visited him at his home and Ali couldn't find his championship belts to show him. Then Plimpton observed Ali struggling to sign his name. He was changing. In September that year, Ali checked into a New York medical center and told reporters, "I'm not suffering. I'm in no pain. It's really nothing I can't live with. But I go to bed, I sleep eight, ten hours, and two hours after I get up, I'm tired and drowsy again. Sometimes I have trembling in my hands. My speech is slurred. People say to me, 'What did you say? I can't understand you.' I'm not scared but my family and friends are scared to death."

In the late 1980s, Gary Smith of *Sports Illustrated*—who had interviewed Ali several times before—went through the process of reintroducing himself to Ali because he thought Ali had forgotten him. Then the former heavyweight champion asked Smith if he wanted to watch him work out. Smith said yes and Ali proceeded to awkwardly struggle to open the gym door, trying to get the key in the lock. He might have still been able to impress on the bags inside, but getting in and then locking up was another matter. By this time, Ali was sometimes drifting off to sleep while at events or even in conversation.

So how much of it was attributable to boxing? "Virtually all of it," Hauser reckoned. And he was not alone. "I know that Lonnie [Ali's wife] didn't want to believe that boxing was the primary cause, but all of the medical records that I saw that were in the late 1990s indicated that boxing was the cause. Stanley Fahn, who was the head of the Movement Disorder Clinic at Columbia Presbyterian Hospital, where Ali was fully evaluated, said boxing was the primary cause. Dennis Pope, who oversaw his care at the UCLA Medical Center, said boxing was the primary cause, and in the late 1990s there was no indication whatsoever of Parkinson's disease."

"Lonnie wanted to believe that he had this bradykinesia, that plasmapheresis was going to treat him because it was caused by creosote poisoning at Deer Lake, and they had this theory and that theory. Now it's possible that in later years, Ali also developed Parkinson's disease. I don't know if he did or not, but certainly boxing was the primary cause and I had all of his medical records and that was clear from studying them."

The physician Rajko Medenica met Ali in 1988 and told the fighter that the slowing of his speech and movement was due to his blood being contaminated with pesticides from his Deer Lake training headquarters so he started having treatment for that. Every three months, Ali would visit the Hilton Head Hospital in South Carolina for "plasmapheresis," which saw his blood removed, filtered through a machine, and then returned to the body—now in unpolluted form. Medenica predicted a complete recovery, which did not happen. Other doctors tested Ali for pesticides and never found any evidence of them.

Of course, the old punch-drunk terminology was rarely used with Ali. Perhaps they thought it was too cruel a label for a man who had given so much and who had awed the world with his brutal elegance.

But there had been too much punishment.

Statistics from CompuBox, which compiled the punch stats from all of Ali's filmed fights, revealed a worrying trend as he continued too long after his best years. CompuBox recorded the blows Ali took and handed out in forty-seven of sixty-one professional contests, and if you add up the punches he took in fights, he was hit 8,877 times.

According to the CompuBox book, *Muhammad Ali: By the Numbers*, he took 1,182 punches in the four fights (two against Spinks, Holmes, and Berbick) after Pacheco walked away.

And, of course, it wasn't just the fights. It was the training camps and the sparring sessions too. Someone who was already damaged goods was becoming more damaged, and even though people in boxing could see it, no one could do anything to stop him finding a way to fight on.

"You can label it any way you want, but Sugar Ray Robinson, Joe Louis, and Muhammad Ali—the three greatest fighters of all time—all fought too long and they all wound up in terrible health with various cognitive issues," continued Hauser. "There's a common denominator in that for anybody who's paying attention."

When Ali turned seventy, daughter Rasheda was interviewed about his health. "We really don't know why he has Parkinson's," she said. "It could have been from boxing but nobody knows yet. That's why it's important to donate time and energy to research, so we can find that out."

But for Ali it was too late. He died on June 3, 2016, at the age of seventy-four. He had been unwell for more than three decades.

✳ ✳ ✳

Years later, several voices could be heard saying Ali should have done more for CTE and that he could have helped the cause of ex-fighters immeasurably had he handled things differently. Some say it was a missed opportunity for boxing; one was fight historian Mike Silver.

"The false narrative with Ali has mostly been foisted with two things: people who are ignorant of the problem and they don't understand it or they're Ali lovers that don't want to believe it," he said. "And his own family, who are really trying to preserve his legacy in the most positive light by saying that Muhammad Ali developed Parkinson's disease, say that he suffered from Parkinson's disease and he would have even got that if he was a bricklayer. That was ridiculous. Now, would he have developed Parkinson's on his own? Possibly. But you cannot tell me, no logical person would tell me or would say that someone who has taken whatever it was he took, and he took some horrific beatings—especially to the head, especially with Shavers—that his brain is not going to be affected by that. In the fifty years I've been a student of boxing, I have never seen a boxer deteriorate as quickly as Muhammad Ali, who by his late forties was basically shuffling, mumbling, and whose handwriting disintegrated. Then, for his family to say that he suffered from Parkinson's . . . that does a disservice to the sport. He's basically boxing's poster-person for brain damage."

Silver believes that Ali's family should have donated his brain for research as does one of the world's leading neurologists, Robert Cantu. He was left conflicted by Ali, respectful of him as an athlete and humanitarian but disappointed he didn't leave his brain behind to be examined. "I admire him greatly, but I do not admire that he did not allow his brain to be studied because I think he was trying to protect boxing and I think that was a mistake," said Cantu. "I think his brain certainly needed to be studied, and I don't know this for a fact so I'm speculating, but I think he made the decision that he wasn't going to let his brain be studied."

Thomas Hauser disagreed that Ali and his family could and should have done more. "No," he countered. "He chose to be an advocate for those suffering from Parkinson's and those fighting Parkinsonism. To Muhammad, by definition if you were advocating for fighters who have CTE, then by definition you were advocating against boxing. Any time somebody talks about all the studies that show an outsized proportion of football players in the United States suffering from CTE, what they are really saying is that football causes brain damage. What's Ali going to do? Get up and say, 'I'm talking the way I am because I boxed for too long? Boxing did this to me?' Well, then the next thing would be, 'Don't box!' And he wasn't prepared to say that. I remember—and I wrote this in one of my later articles—when I finished writing *Muhammad Ali: His Life and Times*, I went out to the farm in Berrien Springs, and Lonnie and I read every word of the manuscript aloud with Muhammad and [Ali's friend] Howard Bingham. I did that for a couple of reasons. Number one, there was some negative stuff about Muhammad in the book and I didn't want him to feel sandbagged when it came out. Number two, I felt that reading the manuscript would elicit additional thoughts from him, which I could incorporate in the book, which in fact happened. And number three, if there was something factually inaccurate in the book, then he could tell me and I could change it. And I remember very clearly, at one point Lonnie was reading a quote from Alex Wallau where Alex, who early on was a producer for ABC Sports and later became president of ABC, said, 'I believe that, even if Ali knew when he started out what his physical condition would be today, he would still do things exactly the same way. He'd still choose to box.' Ali was listening to all this. He sat up straight in his chair and said, 'You bet I would.' There you are."

And lessons were apparently being learned. Ali's daughter, Laila, was one of the sport's finest female fighters. She retired after an unbeaten career of twenty-four wins, looking as immaculate after as she did before. She got out at the right time, and then even wrote a book called *Food for Life* to assist those suffering with chronic illnesses to make healthy food choices. There is also a Muhammad Ali Parkinson Center in Phoenix and a Lonnie and Muhammad Ali Legacy Care Program there.

"Ali preferred to think that boxing was not the cause," said Hauser. "And my sense is because first it tied in with his vanity as a great boxer, and secondly he didn't want to think that boxing—which he loved—would cause something like this. But there's no doubt in my mind that boxing was the primary cause."

As is often the case, there are always dissenting voices. Ali's nearest and dearest might not have held boxing accountable, and neither did his promoter Bob Arum. When asked whether Ali was an example of what can happen to fighters, he said, "Not necessarily. I promoted twenty-five Ali fights and I made him retire after the second Spinks fight and he won the title and then they got him to come back and fight Larry Holmes and Trevor Berbick. I don't think that did him any good. But remember, Ali's family has a history of Parkinson's—his father, his brother . . . and that wasn't because of getting hit in the head. Now, did the boxing and getting hit in the head accelerate it or emphasize it? Probably, but Ali is not a good example of this punch-drunk syndrome. He's not. Ali would have had Parkinson's in any event."

* * *

Meanwhile, Quarry's descent into darkness was as ugly as there's been. The former heavyweight star and golden boy with the looks that made him a Hollywood celebrity, the charisma to charm CEOs and the intelligence to impress them, faded rapidly to black.

One of the first symptoms for Quarry was short-term memory loss. Those close to him thought he may have been overdoing the party life but it was more serious. When *Sports Illustrated* tested him in 1983, the research team found a cavum, enlarged lateral and third ventricles, and possible cortical atrophy. Quarry also scored poorly on several of the tests. He struggled to connect dots, showed some movement problems, although he did not sound "punchy."

Yet despite the findings, he spoke of shaping up and dropping down to cruiserweight to fight for the title. Asked if he would do it again, he said he would. "You damned well know I'd go back into boxing. Yes, sir!" he admitted. Ira Casson told him he shouldn't. Quarry half listened. He took a couple of fights in late 1983 as his weight lowered. He starched an overmatched Lupe Guerra in thirty-two seconds and then went ten rounds to beat James Williams on a majority decision. Then he walked and Quarry should have kept walking, but in 1992, in a Holiday Inn in Aurora, Colorado, the former heavyweight title challenger came back and lost a six-rounder with 3-4-1 Ron Cranmer. Inspired by George Foreman's miraculous comeback in middle age, Quarry was beaten into a pitiful mess by the average Cranmer for a measly $1,050. Quarry lost shards of his teeth that night, needed a hundred or so stitches, and was never the same again.

Of course, many contend that despite the legends Jerry Quarry faced in the ring, the real damage was done in the gym, and mostly inflicted by his brother Mike, a light heavyweight who was world-class in his own right and who teed off on his big brother as he always had something to prove to their megalomaniac father.

Cranmer set off a disastrously bleak period for the Quarrys. In 1995, Jerry told his sister, Janet, "I can feel something wrong in my brain. I don't know what to do."

He was told he had dementia pugilistica and he became frighteningly aware of it. He tried to read up about what was happening. He wondered if he would get better, as though he had a common cold and he was going to shake it. His family watched, powerless to intervene and his mother was heartbroken.

As time went on, he was not allowed to drive and he was picking up a disability allowance of $614 a month. The money from the multiple $200,000 and $400,000 paydays was long gone. It was said he'd earned more than $2 million in total.

It was around this time that his neuropsychologist infamously said, "Jerry Quarry's brain looks like the inside of a grapefruit that has been dropped dozens of times." His brain was getting smaller as cells were dying and, according to Steve Springer, who wrote the devastatingly gripping book on Quarry titled *Hard Luck*, "The doctor likened Jerry's dying brain cells to sugar dissolving in water."

Quarry had a limited life to live out. The inevitability of it all made it even worse.

He moved in with his mother until she couldn't cope, then he moved in with his brother, James, until James couldn't manage. Jerry then went into full-time care. Through that period, the local police had been put on alert that they may find a former boxer roaming the streets not knowing who he was or where he was going and he was escorted home several times. Then things became truly grim.

Pete Hamill, writing for *Esquire*, painted a stark portrait of the former matinee idol. "He needs help shaving, showering, putting on shoes and socks. Soon, probably diapers. His older brother, James, cuts meat into little pieces for him so he won't choke and has to coax him to eat anything except the Apple Cinnamon Cheerios he loves in the morning. Jerry smiles like a kid. Shuffles like an old man now. Slow, slurred speech. Random thoughts snagged on branches in a dying brain. Time blurred. Memories twisted. Voices no one else hears."

Just after turning fifty, he managed to faintly say, "I feel like an old man."

One of his sisters recalled the last time she saw Jerry and said it was as if he was a five-year-old.

On December 28, 1998, Quarry was hospitalized with pneumonia. On January 3, 1999, he suffered a cardiac arrest. Family members asked doctors to remove the life support. There would be no more suffering for Jerry Quarry. He was only fifty-three.

* * *

More sorrow was to come for the Quarry family, however. Kid brother Mike won sixty-two of eighty-two pro fights and followed Jerry into the darkness. Perhaps Mike's decline was accelerated by years of cocaine abuse, but by 2005 he was paranoid, delusional, and aggressive. Eventually he was committed to a psychiatric ward in Brighton Gardens in Yorba Linda, California, and later moved to an assisted-living facility in La Habra. But his body was closing down and in July 2006, it closed for good. Mike was just fifty-five.

The wonderful, teak-tough fighting Quarry boys had fought until the end, but boxing had claimed them both.

Jimmy Quarry, not a fighting sibling, died in 2002. That left one brother, Bobby Quarry, himself a tough slugger back in the 1980s and the youngest of the brood. He retired with ten wins, twelve losses, and two draws and lived in Bakersfield, California, not far from the final resting places of his brothers. There were reports that he had stopped fighting because he was becoming symptomatic back in 1984, after eleven fights, but in 1987 he returned and lost nine of his remaining twelve contests. He was stopped or knocked out in his last four. His final outing was in August 1992.

"I'm doing well," Bobby said in 2018. "I've got a girlfriend. Everything's cool." He maintained his health and, at almost fifty-nine years of age, was just fine. He believed this was because he didn't face the same rigorous amateur schedule that his father had put his brothers Jerry and Mike through.

Bobby was just three when Jerry turned professional and seven when Mike turned over. "It was cool, having brothers like that," he recalled. "I was kind of young so I didn't really understand what it was and then you start appreciating it a lot more as you get older."

As kids, Jerry and Mike learned hard and fast about boxing. Father Jack taught them and he would also adjudicate sparring sessions between the competitive boys. They engaged in hundreds and hundreds of violent seesaw sessions. Jerry was bigger and heavy-handed so Mike, a light heavyweight, took the brunt of it, although Mike could let his hands go because Jerry was so durable.

In *Hard Luck*, the nature of the sessions come to life and Jack is shown imploring them to fight hard and push each other to their limits. "They were very well-known for that," Bobby said. "That book got a little carried away. My dad was not an animal. My dad passed down the only profession he really knew how to hand down and he did a good job. But he wasn't the person who said, 'If you don't have wars with one another I'm not going to help you or I'm not going to take you.' It wasn't to that extent. Jerry, Mike, all of us, we all sparred hard and I sparred with Jerry when he made a comeback in '83, I sparred with Mike probably more than any individual I ever sparred with and, yes, we went at it. That was what we were taught. That was inbred into us. If I hold back in the gym I'm not going to be in the top shape I can be in for the fight."

Bobby continued: "My brothers started boxing at three or four years old and never stopped. I started boxing at three or four but I quit at six or seven and I played my junior high school sports and got into that. They weren't even allowed to play high school sports because they were that good as amateurs. . . . They had an accumulation of blows throughout all their lives. I didn't box from six, seven, until I was seventeen again. They had already had two hundred fights by that time . . . I had twenty-four pro fights, Jerry had sixty-six, Mike had eighty-one or two and that was just pro fights."

There were plenty who would say Bobby was pulled from fighting for his own safety after what happened with Jerry and Mike. But by this time the California commission had allowed him to fight even though he had diminished reflexes in his left arm, something that still tremors to this day. He admitted he didn't want to take any chances after what had happened to his brothers.

"You see, Mike had repercussions when he was still boxing, way back in the '70s," Bobby continued. "Mike's [signs] were more physical— equilibrium, depth perception, dexterity. . . .You wouldn't have noticed but his family did. We knew. Jerry's was more mental. Jerry's mind, we didn't even know he had any problems until about eight or nine years before he passed away. And boom, it was just there. He really couldn't take care of himself."

Grainy YouTube footage exists of Jerry Quarry getting battered by Cranmer at the Holiday Inn, a bout that should never have been allowed, like a lower-rent version of Ali and Berbick.

"That should have never been done," Bobby said. "And of course, Jerry really didn't know that he was not mentally 100 percent at that time, even though he wasn't. He thought he could beat the world, but the people around him should have realized it was an ex-boxer talking the garbage that they always talk. A fighter's the last to realize he don't got it no more."

Did the brothers know the damage was boxing related?

"Oh yeah," Bobby said, before pausing for thought. "Jerry maybe not. Michael knew that he had some mental problems. . . . Mike was coherent enough to realize he wasn't 100 percent, but Jerry's came on so quick when he finally came to notice, that I think 90 percent of the time Jerry didn't realize he was in such a bad way. He would have little windows where he would say, 'I'm not 100 percent' or 'I'm not feeling good,' but he would go right back into the daze. It was sad."

Bobby speaks of both his brothers with great reverence. He was closer to Mike in age and therefore closer to him. But Jerry, who was known as an intelligent man who did crosswords in his down time, was his big brother who became a child again later in life. For Bobby, seeing Jerry lose his smarts was as hard as the physical deterioration.

"In eighth grade you take a high school proficiency test and it places you where you go in your next year of high school and Jerry was in the top 5 percent in the nation," he proudly said. "He got an official letter sending him congratulations. He was a really, really smart man."

And through Jerry's decline he became a figurehead, one of the first ever, of dementia pugilistica. It is not how a relative would like to be remembered, but Bobby is no less proud.

"To an extent," he said, when asked if he preferred everyone remembered the Adonis with the left hook rather than the later version of Jerry. "But if it's helpful to the future fighters and people who are going to be put in the same predicament as him. . . . But nobody wants to be a poster child.

"You know, now with the football players getting the problem and even some of the quarterbacks getting concussions, it's becoming more a point of view with people looking at brain damage and the problems, and now they're wearing different helmets, but boxing is hard because what can you do that protects? Even if you wear a headgear, the use of a headgear is to keep you from getting cut, not to absorb punishment. If you've been hit on headgear you can still get a concussion."

Does he worry about his own health worsening? There have been reports of an Alzheimer's diagnosis and he is already on social security because his shaking left hand means he can't work. Bobby confessed that the left-hand tremors he experiences might be from his time in the sport. "[It's a] possibility," he said. "But I don't think [so]. I think it was due to other causes. I did some things that I shouldn't have done and it came back on me. . . ." Bobby didn't elaborate but maintained he still ran five miles a day and still punched a bag.

"In my opinion, boxing was a job, your duty, and if you wanted to be a fighter you had to be like that," he said. "How many punch-drunk fighters, you know, you talk about punch-drunk fighters back in the old days, they didn't think that this is a person's brain, and it's diminishing there. They didn't really look at it and say, 'This is a person's life and their brain and they're terrorizing it.' They just looked at the heroism of what they're doing."

Bobby bears no ill will toward the sport, though he clearly acknowledges the risks and was deeply moved by what happened to his brothers. He has mixed emotions about boxing but contends it's down to the individual, to fight or not to fight.

"My son is eighteen, he's going to the gym a little bit but I never advocated it to him," says Bobby. "I waited until he got to an age where he wanted to see what it's all about, but I never had him do that. I would not have been to blame for something to happen to him."

But as good as the Quarry boys were, it was the sad fate that befell them that they are renowned for. Before he died, the late Jim Quarry set up The Jerry Quarry Foundation for Pugilistica Dementia in 1995. The charity was designed to help old fighters in need. On the website, Jim wrote, "Jerry Quarry won his most outstanding fight of all. Four years before his death, Jerry helped bring worldwide attention to the dangers of contact sports. Even though we knew that someday he was going to die, it was still a major shock. It will make all of us sit up and recognize that something must be done to make contact sports safer. Jerry was an inspiration to all of us. Jerry never quit. We cannot quit on him."

Jim called for donations to build the Foundation and spoke of new laws that were coming to help boxing. The Quarry name was alive again and Jim gave several interviews. "What we found was there was absolutely no help for fighters who had suffered damage in the ring other than immediate medical help when an injury occurred at a particular moment. There also were no studies to show why some fighters are afflicted, and others, who may have taken as much or more punishment in the ring, are not. Jerry was the first major fighter to go public with his condition. Even Sugar Ray Robinson denied any possibility that his condition could have been brought on by his profession. We started the foundation in 1995 in an effort to help those fighters who faced long-term damage," he told Kent Appell of the website Boxing News 24/7 in 2001.

The dream was to produce pension funds for boxers, help them with care after their careers, and introduce medical facilities for fighters. However, once those goals were seen as unattainable, Jim's focus switched to making the sport safer. He talked of a mandatory three-knockdown rule for a whole fight, not just one round, though Jim admitted he needed a CEO to take the charity further. Then the momentum stopped and Jim died in August 2002. The website remained but it's a dead end. There is no quit in a Quarry but Bobby is the last one standing.

* * *

The paths of Muhammad Ali and Jerry Quarry crossed twice. They went their separate ways but were linked by their health problems in later years. Ali pledged to the world that he had Parkinson's syndrome and his family ran with that. Quarry's family confessed to dementia pugilistica. But for many, Quarry and Ali were poster boys for CTE.

For what it's worth, Randall Cobb—who would later say boxing made him a prostitute, only he sold his "blood rather than his ass"—showed no signs of brain damage in the *Sports Illustrated* investigation or indeed later on. Yes, he'd been annihilated in the Holmes fight and he may have been a brawler, but he'd had just twenty-three pro bouts, had knocked over a load of opponents, and he hadn't fought as an amateur. "It can be concluded that the cumulative effects of his short career in the ring have not made a mark—not yet, maybe never," read the report.

Mark Pacheco was twenty-three at the time and he had been boxing since he was four. He thought he'd had around two hundred amateur fights and he'd lost eleven times in the pros, admitting he'd been hurt on a few occasions. After deciding to call it a day he never fought again.

Casson, the chief medical voice in the *Sports Illustrated* piece, implored both communities, medical and boxing, to do more research and tests on fighters to make the sport safer. CT scans and full neurological exams were not cost-effective, and if anything showed on a CT scan it was too late, but neurological tests could help. And Casson didn't want to waste time, either. "Let's start now," he said. "Before another generation of fighters comes through."

Cleveland radiologist Ronald Ross, who *Sports Illustrated* also called upon, was similarly concerned that the sport was not taking their findings seriously. "The big people in boxing haven't commented," he said. "Who's going to pay for these longer studies? What's being done? I'm afraid everything's going to die down."

People still recall that *Sports Illustrated* piece as one of the most important on the subject, but it went nowhere.

6
Rusting Gold

BAD MEMORIES FROM
A MAGNIFICENT ERA

The heavyweight division in the 1970s is remembered romantically as the sport's peak. They were halcyon days when the best fought the best several times over, and the talent pool was ocean deep.

They said they were "Champions Forever," but Muhammad Ali, George Foreman, Joe Frazier, Ken Norton, and Larry Holmes had a strong supporting cast that allowed their brutally colorful generation to be referred to as *the* Golden Era of heavyweight boxing. Through the 1960s and 1970s, the roster included Floyd Patterson, Earnie Shavers, Jerry Quarry, Oscar Bonavena, Jimmy Young, George Chuvalo, Duane Bobick, Jimmy Ellis, Ernie Terrell, Cleveland Williams, Scott LeDoux, Ron Lyle, Sonny Liston, Chuck Wepner, and others. They beat the hell out of each another, and it's subsequently damning to see what became of so many of them.

Later in the life of Ali's friend, old foe, and sparring partner Jimmy Ellis, stories circulated that his memory was fading. He needed to be reminded of who he was and where he lived. He also had to be routinely told that his wife, Mary, had died, causing fresh heartbreak each time he heard the news. Those looking after Ellis threw a protective cloak over him and refused to let him do interviews because his health was so bad. Then, after he died, his brother Jerry confirmed he had been treated for Alzheimer's.

While another Ali opponent, Joe Frazier, succumbed to liver failure, dying in a hospice in 2011, there had been a mental and physical degeneration for years that saw his words slurred and his mind muddled.

Many felt George Chuvalo was the one who had come out unscathed, although he was not always so confident. Ninety-three fights. Twenty years. "I blocked a lot of those," he said, when asked about all the blows he took. He also credited neck exercises with building a shock absorber that could withstand the heaviest of punches.

"If you have a neck like a stack of dimes you can know that guy's getting knocked out," he said. "I used to stand on my head a lot. A lot of people don't understand that fighters pay scant attention to the punch-absorbing muscles. In football, you do a lot of it in your shoulders. Their muscles are trained to dish out punishment and absorb impact. But very few fighters spend time on muscles to absorb punishment. I used to spend a lot of time on it. It's important. I also think physiologically, certain people have things [going] for them. I have a big jaw and a short neck."

And Chuvalo did take a lot of abuse, regardless of his protestations of being better defensively than he was given credit for. "One man's meat is another man's poison," he said of getting out and still being articulate, bright, and charismatic. "Before I started fighting, I used to stutter and couldn't remember a goddamn thing. Now I remember everything and don't stutter at all. I'm lucky that way. . . . By the way, Chuck Wepner is speaking pretty good and so did [Rocky] Marciano and so did Jack Dempsey in retirement."

Chuvalo continued: "I look at Carl 'Bobo' Olson and some of these guys and he never had a mark on him after a fight. He couldn't even talk later in life. But you never know how you're going to be in retirement. Like today I'm all right—who knows how I will be tomorrow. Look at Floyd Patterson [who Chuvalo shared a vicious Fight of the Year with in 1965]. He was okay until a few years ago. Then, all of a sudden, he couldn't remember a thing. Ingemar Johansson, they tell me his wife had to show him her driving license so he could recognize her."

Around ten years after Chuvalo said that, about the time of his eight-ieth birthday, a feature on the *Toronto Star* website looked behind the scenes of a celebration to mark the milestone and he "was starting to slip away."

"After a pro career of ninety-three fights and innumerable blows to the head, the legendary boxer has 'significant cognitive impairment.'" That was according to a medical assessment filed amid family acrimony. The story went on to say that he had gotten lost driving home. Chuvalo was the subject of a custody feud between his wife and his children from a previous marriage. His son, Mitch, said, in a sworn 2015 statement to act as his dad's litigation guardian, that Chuvalo's memory had ebbed "to the point where my father can no longer be trusted to govern his affairs."

Everyone thought Chuvalo had come out unscathed. He had been in with them all, never dropped, never tasted the canvas, was still standing, in great health in retirement, a success despite several personal tragedies that befell him including the suicides and drug overdoses of two sons and the suicide of his first wife. His ability to survive, to stay standing through it all, was something to boast about. He was hit by the heaviest punchers of a generation hundreds of times, his brain rattled repeatedly, but he never had any sign of damage, let alone destruction. Little did anyone know that it had just taken longer for the disease to take hold before closing Chuvalo down, starting from the brain and working its way out from there.

His wife, Joanne, said medical professionals had warned her that Chuvalo's behavior could change "as his symptoms of head trauma worsen." Those who examined Chuvalo as part of the extremely messy custody proceedings could not say for sure that boxing was responsible for his cognitive slide. However, they knew his profession and were aware of his reputation.

With the confusion of a tug-of-war over him, he didn't know if he was coming or going. As *Boxing News* editor Matt Christie said, "Bang goes Chuvalo being the go-to example when justifying being punched in the face. He was always the equivalent of the ninety-nine-year-old smoking granddad reference when justifying their habit. Such a shame he's in that state." The last time Christie saw Chuvalo, the Canadian giant's thick jaw hung agape, saliva slipped from the side of his mouth. His open eyes were home to a vacant stare.

Then there was Philadelphia's Jimmy Young. In his fifties and after a career of fighting men like Ali, Shavers, and Norton, he was broke and destitute. He died from a heart attack but, again, the signs of his career were evident for all to see and hear. Young, however, was not a tough brawler like Chuvalo or Quarry, but a skilled, defensive technician. "He was brilliant," historian Bert Sugar used to say. Some labeled Young boring, but the idea, of course, is to hit and not get hit. Dementia did not discriminate. His long-term memory of dates, places, and opponents was impeccable, but his short-term memory was not so good and the drugs certainly didn't help. Young used alcohol and drugs to numb the symptoms but died on February 20, 2005, at Hahnemann University Hospital in Philadelphia. He was fifty-six.

Norton, too, struggled in later life after a terrible car accident in 1986. His motor capacities were greatly reduced, even though he was still a terrific specimen of a man. Yet an article on Deadspin.com in 2012 was headlined, "No One Knows Exactly How Boxing Broke Ken Norton's Brain."

"Ken Norton never fell down in 39 rounds of professional boxing with Muhammad Ali," wrote Hamilton Nolan. "But Ken Norton did fall down on January 23, 2012, while posing for a picture after a press conference at the Lou Ruvo Center for Brain Health in Las Vegas. I saw it happen. Ken Norton, the esteemed special guest at the press luncheon, shuffled to the front of the room amid the Cleveland Clinic doctors and public relations representatives, let go of his walker, and slowly, oh so slowly, tilted backward and fell through the step-and-repeat backdrop. The doctors helped him up. There's not much else they can do for him."

Norton, the heavyweight Adonis of his generation, died a year later.

It is possible the 1986 car wreck—which, after leaving him with a fractured skull, jaw, and leg but no recollection of the event, forcing him to learn to talk again—expedited his symptoms rather than was solely responsible for them. "The ironic part is that the blow to the head [from the crash] affected his speech," his wife Jacquie used to say. "People think it's from boxing, but it's not."

Norton would concur, saying he was left talking "how 98 percent of people expect an ex-fighter to talk." No one knows for sure, but he would be in a minority of fighters from that era who made it through unharmed. A woman defending her man, and her man's sport, is a common theme in the shake-up of deteriorating health in boxing.

Norton never fought Floyd Patterson, but the sharp and articulate Patterson was a nimble heavyweight who carried violence in his fists, doubts in his heart, and not a great deal of resistance in his chin. "They said I was the fighter who got knocked down the most, but I also got up the most," he would say. Patterson was boxing's first two-time heavy-weight champion and later became the chairman of the New York State Athletic Commission. He was well-spoken and smart; a clean and whole-some face of boxing in the state. But all was not as it seemed. Those knock-downs and stoppage defeats at the weighty gloves of Liston, Chuvalo, and Johansson had damaged Patterson's brain.

New York boxing historian Jack Hirsch recalled the day things went terribly wrong. "A boxing promoter named David Meyrowitz also wanted to run MMA shows in New York over the objection of the [New York State Athletic] Commission," Hirsch explained. "He took [the Commission] to court and when Patterson took the stand, he failed to remember the most basic of things. It was embarrassing that he was put into that position. The next day Patterson resigned."

A report of the court hearing in the *New York Post* in 1998 began, "Legendary fighter and boxing czar Floyd Patterson can't remember whom he beat for the heavyweight title, his secretary's name, or boxing's most basic rules, a heartbreaking videotape shows." Patterson was being paid almost $80,000 a year as chairman of the NYSAC but was being protected, blocked from giving interviews to cover his worsening condi-tion. Among the things he failed to recall under oath were that contests were no longer fought over fifteen rounds but twelve, where he won the heavyweight crown for the first time, and who preceded him as chairman of the NYSAC. In an attempt to answer that question Patterson rum-maged through his pockets looking for a rehearsed response only to find his pockets empty. He blamed the whole thing on a lack of sleep, but dementia had taken hold and his health rapidly declined. Someone said that, as the years went by, he lost his mind. He died eight years after that hearing, aged seventy-one, from Alzheimer's and prostate cancer.

Patterson's great rival was Sweden's Ingemar Johansson, who he shared three thrilling tussles with. It was at the climax of their second fight when Johansson, knocked cold by Patterson's leaping left hook (one old foe Chuvalo said could "tear your brains out"), was left with his foot twitching while he was unconscious. Johansson died in 2009, three years after Patterson. For his last six years he was cared for in a home, being treated for Alzheimer's. His cause of death was listed as pneumonia but he had been terribly unwell and was unable to travel to his induction in New York's International Boxing Hall of Fame in 2002. Johansson had been a success after boxing, investing wisely in Sweden, where he was a national hero.

Chicago's Ernie Terrell, a former WBA champion who faced Ali and Chuvalo, also did well for himself. He ran a corporate janitorial business with hundreds of employees, serving businesses, schools, and police precincts. He was an old-fashioned man with traditional values who enjoyed singing. When he died in 2014, at the age of seventy-five, his sister Lovie Mickens said he had dementia.

For decades after he retired in 1973, Terrell was absolutely fine. Then he was not.

Scott LeDoux's fellow Minnesotan Duane Bobick, who fought in the 1972 Munich Olympics, didn't live up to his hype as a pro, eventually getting starched in one gruesome round by Norton. In a comparatively short career spanning six years he fought fifty-two times, winning forty-eight (forty-one by stoppage) and losing four. He was halted in all four losses.

"Boxing was big back in the '70s and there wasn't a lot of knowledge on the effects of being punched in the head over and over again," Bobick's wife, Deb, said. "He never knew years later he would suffer from pugilistic dementia or CTE." In 2011, Bobick told the *Morrison County Record*, "I'm not sure I would have gone into boxing back then if I would have known all the effects of head trauma that I know today, but I don't regret the experience, intense training, and discipline I learned from the sport." By 2018, Bobick—who was born in 1950—was living in a hospice and couldn't recognize Deb or his children.

German southpaw Karl Mildenberger, who fought sixty-two times between 1958 and 1968, facing the likes of Ali, Henry Cooper, Eddie Machen, and Leotis Martin, got out before it was too late, he thought. He lost his European title to Cooper but by then had already decided to call it quits. "If I had retained the title, I would have relinquished it," he said at the time. "Win, lose, or draw, I would have retired anyway. This was the end. I was unharmed. No terrible things had happened to me." He went downhill years later and in 2017 was in awful condition. He died in a hospice in October 2018; the Federation of German Professional Boxers didn't list the cause.

Of all the aforementioned heavyweights, no one, in many ways, was the success story that George Foreman was. His grilling machine sold millions of units worldwide. A champion in two different eras, he had a successful post-fight career as a TV analyst. More than that, he had his health. Aged sixty-nine and as sharp as when he was a young man destroying contenders and champions more than four decades earlier, he had his own theory behind the demise of so many of his contemporaries. Foreman believed boxing was not what had caused such savage deterioration, but the combination of alcohol and/or drugs with fighting spelled trouble for combatants. "I've even talked to my children about this and if you want to be such an athlete, you have to dedicate your life fully to it," Foreman said, referring to sons and daughters who boxed as amateurs and professionals. "You could not and cannot deviate and be a regular guy . . . no drugs, no alcohol whatsoever because even some of the finest prescriptions that are given to human beings, they say do not use alcohol while you're taking these things. Some of these drugs can heal you, but if you feed drugs with alcohol it can destroy you. All of the boxers who had a tendency to use alcohol along with boxing have all faced the same fate; you're going to have some brain injuries. You can't have them both. You can't do it."

Foreman has been a teetotaler since the age of seventeen. He once saw his idol, former American football player Jim Brown, in a commercial telling him that if he wanted to be a great athlete, he couldn't smoke or drink. Foreman listened. "And I did smoke, and I did drink alcohol but I said, 'I'm going to be a boxer' and I stopped all the above and I never went back. And in the ten years I was out of boxing, I didn't even have a sip of wine. I didn't do anything. The brain stayed intact but I knew others who did drink and did do differently and they were different. I looked at them and I thought, 'Uh oh. There's going to be trouble.' And I don't think it's as much the boxing as mixing the two together."

Foreman felt it was an area where young fighters needed education, about living a healthy life away from the ring not only benefiting one's fighting career but helping them in retirement too. Because Foreman was not blind to what happened to Ali, Frazier, Quarry, Terrell, Ellis, Chuvalo, Young, and the others. "When I've gone to some of the Boxing Hall of Fame presentations, I've run into a lot of these guys and I see what you're talking about and I don't like it. But the fact is they were never told; they were never educated. They all thought that you could celebrate with champagne after you become champion and you can't. You've got to celebrate with Kool-Aid and water."

Foreman continued: "I spent many years with Archie Moore, who was the light-heavyweight champion of the world. We called him Teacher Moore because he'd say, 'No, you shouldn't say or do this.' He'd correct your English. He'd correct your behavior and there were no ill effects at all with Archie Moore and he had more than two hundred fights."

Some of the fighters Foreman fought he has since met shuffling and slurring at award dinners, autograph signings, and galas. Does he feel responsible for helping wreak havoc on those men later in their lives? "It's a two-edged sword," he began, having paused for thought. "You cannot feel compassion without feeling a bit of guilt. Even today someone asked me about Muhammad and some of the damage I'd caused and I say there's not been a day in my life in the last twenty-five years that I haven't felt guilt about even laying my hands on Muhammad Ali. I don't know why but there's always been guilt."

Foreman had heard of Chuvalo's deterioration. He stopped the big Canadian after three one-sided sessions back in 1970 in Madison Square Garden. No, he did not put him down, but he landed booming, bruising blows. "George Chuvalo is not a young man," Foreman explained, when asked why it had taken so long for him to go downhill. "Once you hit a certain age and you cash your social security, things happen to people and things can change. I don't worry about it as you age; it's the young guys I worry about."

Those coming through the ranks may have more people looking out for them than either Foreman or Chuvalo did. Research and knowledge of brain injuries is improving, but still those who move into a cold emptiness when the sport spits them back out need help, particularly if they have been damaged. Foreman maintained that it begins with teaching them how to live cleanly and the importance of it. He insisted it was not an argument he mounted because he is a religious man, a minister in Texas. "It's not about religion or good behavior; it's just that they cannot be mixed," he went on. "No one is brave enough to say, 'Hey son, you want to be a boxer? You cannot smoke or drink. You cannot do these things.' There should be an exclamation mark. If not, we should all bear the responsibility of taking care of these guys once these things happen. Literally billions of dollars have been earned through the Mike Tysons, the Holyfields. . . . Some of that money should be channeled to take care of these injuries that people suffer. Even now Anthony Joshua, Deontay Wilder, Floyd Mayweather . . . these guys have generated billions and a portion of that should be set aside to aid all of us one day."

Foreman may not have the most scientific reasoning behind his beliefs, but he has seen enough old fighters over the years to make up his own mind. There was another fearsome heavyweight of the era, Earnie Shavers who was frequently crowned the hardest-hitting heavyweight of all time, the man who hurt Ali and floored Holmes but was unable to finish either. He agreed with Foreman that a wholesome lifestyle outside the ring was likely to help a fighter's longevity after they hung the gloves up.

Shavers had eighty-nine pro fights but said he was never concussed despite sharing some almighty battles and getting stopped or knocked out seven times. That only served to allow one to believe that concussions just were not checked for or talked about at the time. He was at the mercy of a fierce one-round beating by Jerry Quarry, and Ron Lyle detonated a thunderous right hand that left him defenseless on the ropes, where his unprotected head was in line for even more punishment before he finally pitched face-first on the canvas and was counted out by the referee. Against Randall "Tex" Cobb, the thirty-six-year-old was exhausted (he'd also recently had an operation on a detached retina), and commentator Don Dunphy said he had taken "a frightful beating" over the eight rounds it lasted.

Still, Shavers was doing okay later in life. "I agree a thousand percent," he said when asked of Foreman's clean-living theory. "Alcohol is never pretty. Drugs, alcohol, smoking, it will affect you over a period of time and I agree with George. I took care of myself since I was twelve years old. I never drank. Well the worst thing I ever did in my life was after I knocked Jimmy Ellis out they gave me a party and I took two glasses of champagne. I got drunk and I never drank again. I took care of myself and I take care of myself even today. I'm seventy-three years old and I'm in very good health. I have no problems remembering things. I'm working so I'm happy. The key to it is taking care of yourself. If you take too many punches and you don't take care of yourself, it will affect you, but I did the punching so it didn't affect me."

Yet there is one man who had years of life as a rock star during years of taking heavyweight hits to disprove the Foreman concept that Shavers had also adopted. Chuck Wepner was stopped in three rounds by Big George in 1969, mauled in nine by Sonny Liston, and whipped by Muhammad Ali in the fifteenth round, albeit after controversially putting

"The Greatest" on his backside. Ali claimed Wepner stood on his foot and pushed him. Wepner contended it was a body shot. Regardless, the result was never in doubt. It was during that unlikely 1975 showcase against Ali—with a young Sylvester Stallone sitting in the crowd—that the young actor nicknamed "Sly" was inspired to write the script for the original *Rocky* movie. Wepner was Rocky; Ali was Stallone's Apollo Creed.

"The Bayonne Bleeder" was a known tough guy, a brawler who was durable as long as the skin around his eyes held up. He lacked natural talent but made up for it with a hoodlum's charm and his ability to graft. In 2018, aged seventy-nine, Wepner was still going and felt Foreman's analysis was wide from the mark. "I partied hard," he argued. "I partied more than most and I dabbled in a little of everything, but I was so well conditioned. I trained hard and I'm very lucky. I'm one of the lucky ones, and I see some of the guys from my era and even way after my era that are hurt—and it's just the luck of the draw, I think."

The hidden damage caught up to so many of his fellow 1970s heavy-weights. "I think it's been going on for a long time but years ago it wasn't diagnosed," he continued. "It is now. It's a problem, definitely. It's a hitting game and if you know that going in you understand that, like most sports, but boxing is much more prevalent because there's no headgear or anything in a fight. It's something that's been happening a long time and it's going to continue, but they're a lot more careful now. I mean, when I was boxing, you figure I had 328 stitches, nine broken noses, [ruptured] both eardrums, and nowadays you get a cut that requires two stitches and they're stopping the fight. It's a completely different game these days. They're much more careful about stuff like that.

"It catches up to you later on," he said of the accumulated punishment. "I'm one of the lucky guys around, I guess. Hey, I had fifty-two pro fights and over fifty amateur fights in the ring and I'm still okay. I'm still working. I'm still on top of my game. Right now I'm having a little problem with rectal cancer—I've had it for about a year but I'm pretty sure I've come out of that too. They tell me I'm cancer free. I had radiation. I had chemo and everything else so I'm one of the lucky ones. But for me, it all comes down to physical fitness. I trained hard when I fought because I knew I didn't have the talent a lot of these other guys had. I had to train hard to win on attrition. Some of these guys might not train as hard and when they get hit, those blows have a bigger effect."

Did Wepner worry about it catching up to him? "Well I'm seventy-nine years old," he continued. "I'm not worried about getting old or hurt because I am old and I was hurt! But I've worked my way through it. It's just something that you can't worry about. If you're going to be a fighter and you're going to go in the ring worried about getting hurt in any bout you shouldn't be fighting because you're going to get hurt."

So, unlike Foreman, Wepner did not believe it was a concoction of drugs, alcohol, and fast living combined with punishment; it was the sport. Boxing was the link. "Oh yeah, definitely. It's a much tougher game," he explained. "Football, baseball, basketball . . . well, football especially, you got eleven guys and you're substituting in and out and you're wearing shoulder pads, helmets, and all that and in boxing you're just putting on trunks and gloves and you go in there and bang it out. I just think boxing is probably the toughest sport of all of them as far as getting hurt goes."

Yet so many of Wepner's colleagues came out of it far worse than he did, from a time that is remembered with a warm nostalgia, back when boxing was boxing. "The era that I was in . . . you got the greatest heavyweights of all time. When I was ranked in the top ten in the world, we had Foreman, we had Frazier, we had Muhammad Ali, we had Terrell, Bonavena, Quarry, myself. . . . That was the Golden Era of heavyweight boxing."

Of course, some of the heavyweights of Wepner's time did not make it to the age where their hard career inside the ropes might have played a role in their demise. Sonny Liston died suspiciously at the age of thirty-eight, whether it was an accident, he was murdered, or he committed suicide, while Cleveland Williams was killed in a hit-and-run accident in 1999 at the age of sixty-six.

Other heavyweight stalwarts of the 1960s and 1970s included Eddie Machen and Zora Folley. Machen died while sleepwalking, at the age of forty, while Folley's death was ruled accidental if mysterious. He had been in a motel with a married couple and another woman and was fooling around on the edge of the pool. He was either pushed or fell into the water innocuously enough, apparently, but died from his injuries. There were said to be several bumps to the head when the body was checked, but neither the autopsy nor police reports were made public. He, too, was forty.

Decades have passed since the Golden Era. Not many of those TV darlings of the time are still alive, though Foreman, Shavers, and Wepner have managed to hang onto their health into old age. Foreman and

Shavers were the two known for inflicting the most damage and achieving so many early finishes courtesy of their power—power that, in some way, might have brought about the decline in their common opponents.

There were plenty more heavyweights of the era who did not make it to the top of the pile, but they too suffered with poor health after boxing. Later in life, fringe contenders like Donnie Fleeman and Alex Miteff lost their memories and their bodies started to close down. In 2010, former 1960s contender Fleeman told a journalist to come to his house to do an interview. By the time the journalist got there, Fleeman had forgotten. A year or so earlier, Miteff had been found hardly able to talk or move in a hospice in New York, though he tried his hardest.

Meanwhile, Ali's debut opponent, Tunney Hunsaker, who was put in a coma in his last professional fight, suffered the effects of it for the rest of his days before losing his battle with Alzheimer's at seventy-four.

So of those from that Golden Era of heavyweights, the following died from or with symptoms of neurological problems:
• Muhammad Ali (aged 74)
• Jimmy Ellis (aged 74)
• Joe Frazier (aged 67)
• Ingemar Johansson (aged 76)
• Scott LeDoux (aged 62)
• Jerry Quarry (aged 53)
• Floyd Patterson (aged 71)
• Ernie Terrell (aged 75)
• Jimmy Young (aged 56)

They left fans and historians with memories of a Golden Era, but each of them descended—eventually—into a far darker place. Champions forever? Too many clung on to our respect while losing their dignity. Too many signed autographs while unable to write with clarity. Too many posed for pictures without being able to stand steadily. Too many broke the hearts of fans who managed to meet them. They were no longer the supermen but beaten-up old men on a scrap heap that boxing refused to acknowledge or help.

But not Foreman. Somehow not Big George. He remained certain boxing will not get him. Will he struggle as the years go on? "No," he said, resolutely. "Not from boxing. Not at all from boxing."

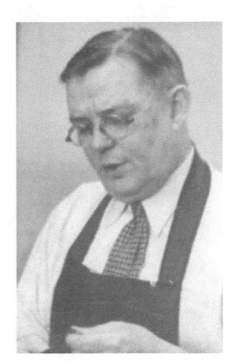

Harrison Martland wrote the paper "Punch Drunk" in 1928 and was the first man to medically coin the phrase. *Rutgers University*

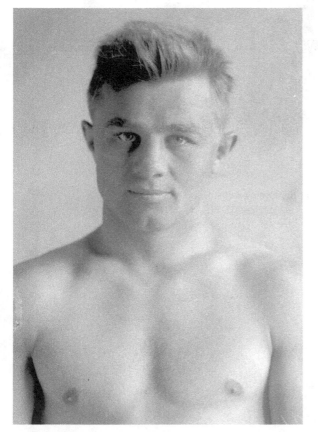

Billy Papke, "The Illinois Thunderbolt," was a brilliant middleweight boxer. In 1936 he killed his wife, Edna, and then committed suicide. *Steve Lott/Boxing Hall of Fame*

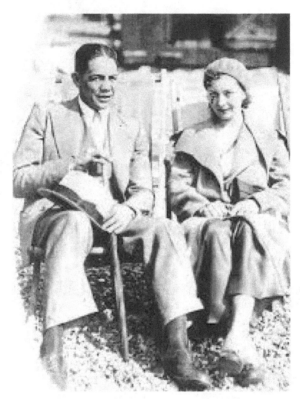

Del Fontaine took his fair share of punishment in the
ring. He murdered his girlfriend, Hilda Meeks, and
his defense claimed he was "punch drunk."

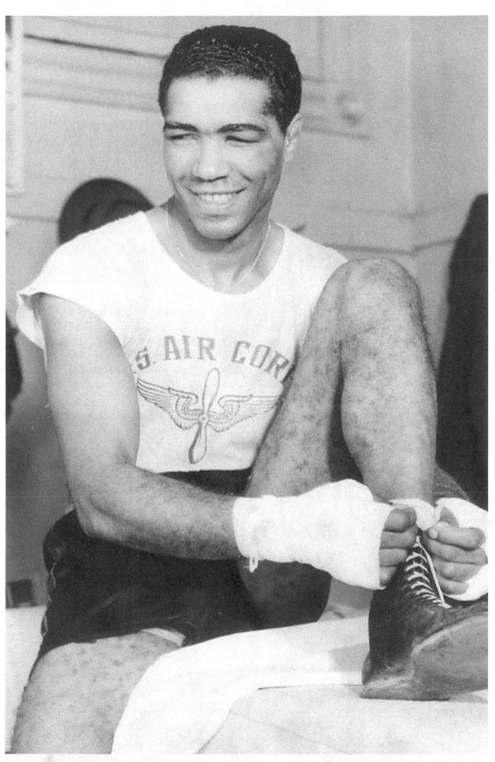

Cocoa Kid, aka Herbert Lewis Hardwick, was diagnosed with dementia pugilistica and discharged from the Navy but continued to box. *Boxing News*

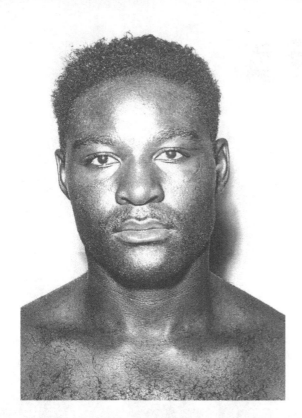

Ezzard Charles was a world champion at light-heavyweight and heavyweight. In the 1970s he was confined to a wheelchair and used as the focal point of a nationwide commercial for muscular dystrophy. *Boxing News*

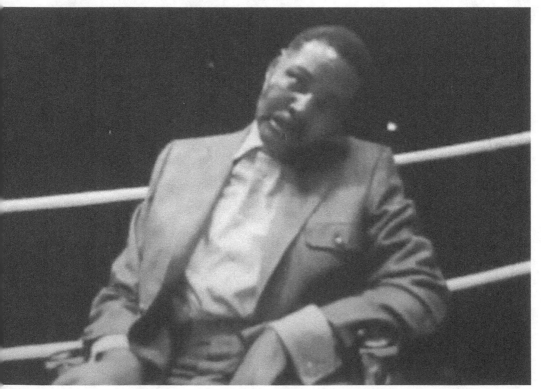

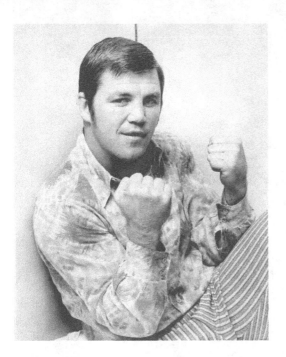

The Quarry brothers, Jerry (left) and Mike, fought hard and legend has it that they sparred one another even harder. Both would suffer tragic declines. *Boxing News*

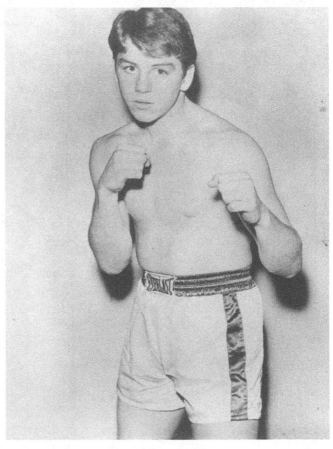

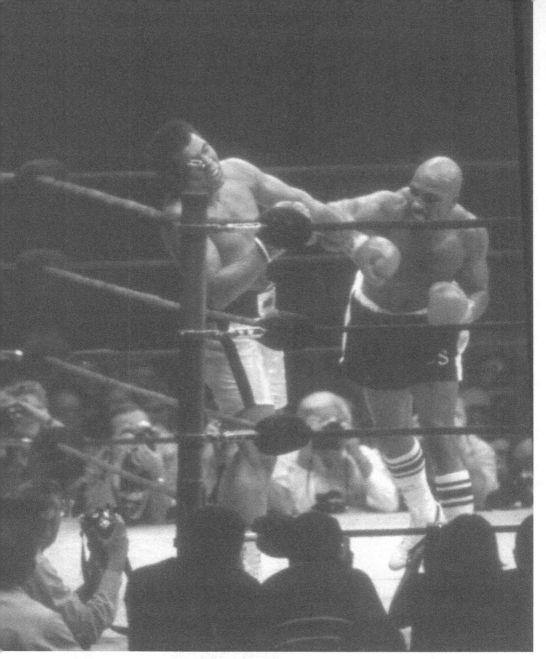

Many believe Muhammad Ali's struggle with the ferocious Earnie Shavers was a fight too far. Ali won, but he fought four more times. *Steve Lott/Boxing Hall of Fame*

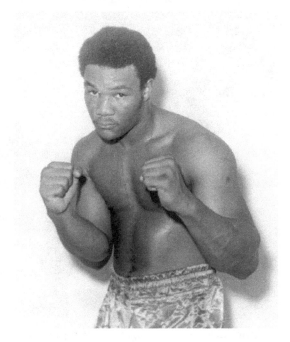

George Foreman had two successful careers in the ring and remains in great health in his seventies. He says it's because he lived a clean life away from the ring. *Boxing News/International Boxing Hall of Fame*

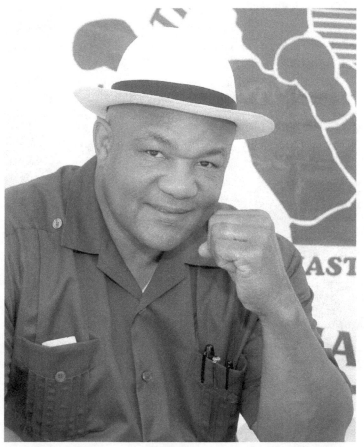

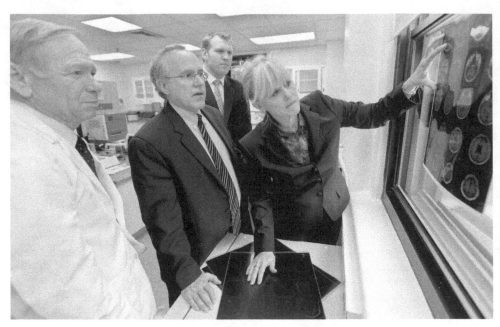

Dr. Ann McKee assesses slides with (left to right) Dr. Robert Cantu, Dr. Robert Stern, and Chris Nowinski. *Concussion Legacy Foundation*

Many believe Meldrick Taylor was not the same fighter after losing to Julio Cesar Chavez. He would have more wins, but fought on too long. *Getty Images*

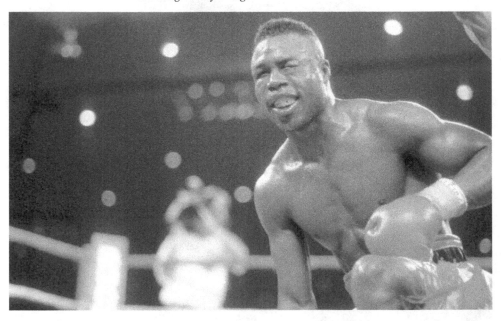

7
Concussion

THE NFL DENIED A CRISIS
BOXING IGNORES

I t was winter in Boston. The orange and yellow of the leaves in Massachusetts had begun to fade, creating a deep auburn blanket beneath rows of trees. Ann McKee was heading to the Veterans Administration Hospital, another day at the office, but there was a spring in her step. She was a neuropathologist for the Alzheimer's disease brain bank, and she'd heard about the death of a former boxer named Paul Pender. Pender, a former world middleweight champion in the 1960s, had wound up as an inpatient at the VA and his death had caused a stir. He'd defeated, among others, Sugar Ray Robinson, Carmen Basilio, Ralph Jones, and Terry Downes in a comparatively brief career of forty wins, six losses, and two draws. He was seventy-two when he died on December 1, 2003, but family and friends had noticed behavioral changes in his fifties, perhaps even earlier. There was forgetfulness, bursts of aggression, and a gradual decline in health.

"Something's wrong with me," he told his wife, Rose. But Pender, a bright, articulate man, didn't know what. He couldn't understand why he wasn't remembering appointments. He was finally admitted to the VA Hospital after Rose had spent years looking after him at home. He died eighteen months later and his widow donated his brain to research in an extraordinary gesture and pivotal moment in boxing history.

"We removed the brain and our process is to fix half and freeze half," said McKee. "You can't really tell from looking at the brain immediately upon removal what's going on, you have to do a microscopic exam to be sure, but you could tell it was small. It appeared to have some damage, particularly in the central areas of the brain, but I wasn't sure what it was. I knew the clinicians who had seen him during his life thought it was Alzheimer's disease and in speaking to them about it—in retrospect now—they said they didn't consider that his neurodegeneration and dementia would be due to boxing because he retired at the age of thirty-two and became symptomatic in his mid-fifties. He was hospitalized in his sixties and died in his early seventies. They felt that there'd been too long a lag period to explain his decline from boxing."

McKee had seen a lot of brains over the previous two decades, but she'd not seen anything like Pender's. She'd always had a fascination with brain diseases and tau protein, something that kills brain cells. She'd been on various medical boards involved with Parkinson's, Alzheimer's, and dementia, and she had studied degenerations. Now, almost twenty years later, she remembered the day in 2003 clearly. It was the day she came face-to-face with CTE.

McKee expected to see Alzheimer's, given Pender's diagnosis. "And the first thing I saw was that he had absolutely no beta amyloid in his brain, and for the diagnosis of Alzheimer's disease you need lots of beta amyloid and in the form of neuritic plaques. He had none. That took that diagnosis off the table. Looking at [his brain] under the microscope, he had the most extraordinary pattern of tau that I had ever seen. It was a pattern of pathology I'd never seen before. It was really curious because it circled around blood vessels, it was extremely patchy, it involved patches of the nervous system that are relatively spared in Alzheimer's disease . . . it was like an extreme form of a tauopathy. I started looking up papers of CTE and noticed that in the 1990s there had been two reports of this perivascular tau pattern; one was in an autistic woman who died at the age of twenty-four, who was thought to have dementia pugilistica on the basis of head-banging, and I'd also seen a report of several young boxers in their twenties, a rugby player and an epileptic with poorly controlled seizures with that pattern of tau pathology. I was starting to think this perivascular, this accentuation around the blood vessels, this patchy distribution was a characteristic of CTE and I was fascinated."

McKee continued: "If you're studying something for decades and then you see a pattern that's wildly different, that's exciting, and you're also curious about it, so I became curious to find other boxers. I was able to go through the VA records and found a couple and it seemed they had the same disease, but I was having trouble getting more brains."

It wasn't long before an influx was coming her way, because, in Pittsburgh, neurologist Bennet Omalu was conducting his own research. Omalu examined the brain that sparked the NFL's concussion crisis in 2002 but his work on Mike Webster wasn't published until it appeared in *Neurosurgery* in 2005 in a paper titled "Chronic Traumatic Encephalopathy in a National Football League Player." Omalu was a Nigerian doctor who knew nothing about American football or Webster, a Hall of Fame Pittsburgh Steeler. What Omalu discovered was incredible. He described his findings as "abnormal accumulations of protein," and it was the first documented case of CTE in an NFL football player.

Webster was fifty when he died on September 24, 2002. He was classified as disabled and suffered with amnesia, depression, and dementia. The picture history painted of the legendary NFL gridiron star was stark. He lost his fortune and got divorced. He isolated himself. He was so broke that he lived in his car and in so much pain that he had to taser himself to sleep. He glued his teeth back in if they came out, and he finally succumbed to a heart attack.

Then came Terry Long, a Pittsburgh teammate of Webster who played guard and was only forty-five when he died. Then Andre Waters, a former Philadelphia Eagle safety, followed. He was forty-four. Then there was another former Steeler, Justin Strzelczyk, thirty-six, who played tackle. All of them had CTE.

Long, who had a lengthy legal history of charges from fraud to arson to firearm possession, committed suicide in 2005 when he downed a bottle of antifreeze. He had made several attempts on his life and had suffered from a series of psychiatric problems.

Waters, who coached football in retirement, shot himself in the head. Although he was forty-four, his brain tissue, according to Omalu, was "that of an eighty-year-old man with Alzheimer's disease, caused or hastened by the numerous concussions Waters sustained playing football."

Strzelczyk also had issues. There were charges of DUIs and firearm possessions and when he died, in 2006, his car was travelling at ninety miles per hour into oncoming traffic as he tried to escape police. Some thought an autopsy would show he was high on drugs or alcohol, but he wasn't. It did, however, reveal that he was brain damaged from years of football.

Webster had retired from football in 1990, the same year a brilliant "Terrible" Terry Norris obliterated the feared John "The Beast" Mugabi for the WBC's world junior-middleweight title. Norris would box until 1998, losing his final three fights before admitting it was over. Then came not only a boxing wilderness but a wilderness he faced while damaged severely from the sport. He was only thirty-one but the future Hall of Famer was "shot" or "gone." He'd made big money. That was gone, too.

"I think fighters in general are not prepared for what comes after boxing," said veteran Showtime announcer Steve Farhood. "And if you add the element of potential brain trauma or CTE or something as serious as that, then they're really unprepared, and boxing . . . does nothing to help them. I also think that the fact that we don't discuss this issue more is emblematic of the fact that a lot of people in boxing, and perhaps boxing as a sport, tends to treat its fighters as disposable commodities. They are warriors as long as they can fight, and when they can no longer fight at that level, they're useless to a lot of people. That's very sad but I don't think it's being overstated."

Norris didn't have the best ability to take a punch, suffered some brutal knockouts, and one loss came at the violent fists of Julian Jackson. Farhood said he's seen those knockouts and witnessed a fighter leave the ring under his own steam but wondered whether such blows will take effect in twenty or thirty years.

"When I see a knockout like that, unfortunately that's what comes to mind," he said. "Then we have a tendency, when a fighter retires after a long and tough career, to say, 'Well, he got out at the right time' or 'Fortunately he seems to have all his faculties.' But what we miss in that situation is where is he going to be in ten or twenty years. There's no guarantee that all will be good."

For Norris it wasn't good. He'd had almost three hundred amateur fights (291-4) and his pro record was 47-9 (31). By 2000, the Nevada State Athletic Commission was telling him it was over because they could hear he wasn't right. "I'm not exaggerating," remembered physician Margaret Goodman, who was then on the commission. "Every one of the commissioners had a tear in his eye, because it was right there staring you in the face what had transpired to this amazing young man. You didn't need a million-dollar study to tell you this young man didn't belong in a boxing ring anymore. Everybody respected Terry so much. To see that happen to such a wonderful boxer and wonderful person was tragic."

Norris's speech became muddled and his memory started to falter. His great wins were being erased from within. By his late forties he could hardly remember them. He became so embarrassed that sometimes he would cry in public. There'd been years of speech therapy and physical therapy to relax his contracting muscles. Was it all worth it? "I would say it was," he said once. "I put my family on the map. I made my dad happy."

One of Norris's best wins came against electric Philadelphian Meldrick Taylor, a 1984 Olympic star who owned some of the fastest hands in boxing but was arguably defined by a heartbreaking final-two-second loss to the great Mexican fighter Julio Cesar Chavez in a twelve-round war. "Meldrick had gone from elite to merely world-class," International Boxing Hall of Fame writer Bernard Fernandez said of what remained of Taylor post-Chavez. "He was bright again but never dazzling, the hurricane that blew at a force ten was now a seven or eight . . . when he fought Terry Norris, that was when he was really exposed as not being the same guy. A few years later, the slurring in his speech was extremely pronounced."

Fernandez continued: "It was sad because he made a good amount of money and he had two attorneys and Main Events had set up an annuity for him where he was going to get paid hundreds of thousands of dollars a year forever. And after he got knocked out by [Crisanto] Espana, he went and looted the annuity. And they said, 'Don't do it, you're going to need it in later years' and he said, 'It's my money,' which it was, but then he had nothing and he became a cliché. He was great but then he had nothing to fall back on. . . . Dr. Goodman said there's no way he should have been allowed to fight with his cognitive tests. If you take a test at school and you get a ninety-eight, you're going to get an A-plus. If passing is seventy and you get right on seventy you're passing but you're not where you were. He was taking some fights at the end for like $2,000. There were people telling Meldrick to stop but he was saying 'I'm passing the tests so I can fight.' I understand that rationale. It's right but it's also wrong."

Farhood covered the brilliant careers of Norris and Taylor, but also witnessed their declines and admitted it's been sad to see boxing take a toll. "Meldrick, while we can't be sure which fights caused his problem, you think of the amount of punishment he took in that first Chavez fight, and you wonder how much that relates to the way he is today," Farhood considered. "You see some of these fighters and they are prime examples, in relation to the fighters before them, they had very few fights, yet they suffered the somewhat inevitable problems former fighters have. Part of the outrage that we hear when a fighter does die in the ring is that there's always an outcry, as there should be. But so much of it is often politically motivated, and no one is thinking about Meldrick or the fighters who suffered long-term damage. They talk about the fatalities, that it should be banned, etc., etc., but the fighters suffering the effects that they have to live with for maybe thirty or forty years just don't seem to generate the same amount of attention."

Farhood has seen numerous safety procedures improve during his four decades covering the sport. He was ringside when Willie Classen died in New York in 1979 when they had to hail an ambulance from the street with no oxygen in the venue and no ringside care, but the risk can't be removed entirely. "There's a dark inevitability that things are going to happen and the connection to CTE is hardly surprising," said Farhood.

Boxers had suffered similar fates for decades but then McKee discovered a similar pattern of tau to Pender's in another deceased patient's brain. In fact, in this brain, there was so much tau it could be seen by the naked eye. Under the microscope, scientists could see where neurons had died in several parts of the brain, such as the hippocampus, and there was patchy tau in a number of regions. There was no amyloid beta. The damaged areas could explain things like short-term memory loss and depression. Yet when McKee inquired about the patient's history, she was told the brain damage couldn't have been trauma related. It was just another elderly patient at the VA. There were no stories of world titles and no coulda-been-a-contender tales although when McKee called the patient's family to cross-check, she was told that he had boxed throughout his twenties.

✳ ✳ ✳

Then, in 2008, McKee took a call from Chris Nowinski, founder of an organization called the Concussion Legacy Foundation. Nowinski started the CLF in Boston in 2007 to support athletes, veterans, and anyone affected by concussions or CTE and its aim is to make sports smarter so they are safer for participants. Nowinski was a former Harvard football player and WWE wrestler whose ring moniker was Chris Harvard. He played the part of a righteous but dastardly Ivy Leaguer who would win by any means necessary. But his own career was curtailed after he suffered a series of concussions that left him with lasting symptoms, including terrible headaches. He had met with Dr. Robert Cantu who would forever change Nowinski's outlook about sports and brain injuries as he began a new mission in his life, to live in a world without CTE and to teach concussion safety without compromise. It would all start with research. Nowinski had watched with interest as Omalu made his discoveries, and the two worked with one another briefly when families of deceased football players began donating brains to the foundation to be studied, Nowinski and Omalu fell out and then went through a spell competing for brains and science. But as the NFL made Omalu's life miserable by taking a stance of denial and trying to discredit his work, Nowinski set about trying to find more brains and more answers. Then, with Omalu out of the picture, Nowinski needed a top neuropathologist to examine his findings. With his extraordinary Rolodex, he could reach out to football players, wrestlers, and their families as he had done when he obtained the brain of Chris Benoit, the Canadian "Crippler" who, in 2007, killed himself after murdering his wife and their seven-year-old son. Omalu had discovered CTE "in all regions" of Benoit's brain.

McKee didn't need to dwell on the Nowinski offer. She was in. "Of course, I jumped at the chance because I was interested in trauma and the effects in the brain," she remembered. Then, she went on:

> "Also I was a huge football fan so I was very excited by the possibility. I'd been a football fan for many years and I've been a neuroscientist

since I started neurology in '81 and I never thought they were getting any bad brain injuries. Even though I was aware of neurological deterioration I just, as a fan, did not think they were endangering their brain. You can't see it, there's no blood, there's no pain, so when I looked at the first football player—[Houston Oilers linebacker] John Grimsley in February of 2008—I was blown away. I saw the same thing I saw in Paul Pender. Again, no beta amyloid, he's forty-five, almost thirty years younger than Paul when he dies, and for me to see that kind of neurodegeneration in the brain of a forty-five-year-old is unheard of. I immediately talked to my brother, who is also a doctor. We had sort of shoptalked at home about football and he was a family doctor so he was seeing some former teammates and some coaches and wondering if there was something in football that was causing some sort of neurologic decline. I showed it to Charles and we both said, 'We've got to tell people. We need to tell the NFL. The NFL needs to understand that this is happening to their players.' And I thought naively that they would become very concerned and want to do everything in their power to prevent this or to understand it, and it was a few months later, I published my first paper in 2009 where I reported all of the cases of CTE in literature [forty-five in all, and just a few years later she would update with a further sixty-eight] and I reported two boxers and our first football player [Grimsley] and that was in September. In November I was asked to present my findings in front of the NFL's Mild TBI [Traumatic Brain Injury] Committee at the time. The person who asked me was Ira Casson—he's well-known now as an ardent denier of CTE, so I was nervous about going. They asked me to go by myself and I was thinking I would be overpowered in a room of all NFL representatives. They did invite a few other doctors and I spoke to Chris [Nowinski] about it and he said, 'Why don't I come too?' and I asked them and they said no, and then I said the only way I can come is if Chris comes, and they came back and said 'Well, he can come but he can't say anything. He can only observe.' So we went and presented to the NFL."

New York neurologist Casson, by the way, was the same scientist called upon by *Sports Illustrated* as the expert in their 1983 piece "Too Many Punches, Too Little Concern." He'd examined Muhammad Ali's

CT scans and determined through his own work that fighters were prone to cavum septum pellucidum, a common feature of CTE.

Through the late 2000s as the co-chair of the NFL's Concussion Committee, Casson presented counterarguments, denying McKee's research and thus protecting the NFL from the avalanche of lawsuits it was readying itself for. He had been seen as a head-injury expert, using neuropsychological tests and state-of-the-art CT scanning technologies to see brain injuries in fighters.

"The boxing community wasn't happy with me," he said, having published "Brain Damage in Modern Boxers" in May of 1984 in which he found 87 percent of eighteen fighters showed "definite evidence" of brain damage. There were several boxing papers around that time, including another by M. Kaste in *The Lancet* in November 1982 that said according to EEG and CT scans that from fourteen fighters, six professionals and eight amateurs, four of the pros and six of the amateurs had "brain injury."

To say the NFL was skeptical of McKee was an understatement. Despite her breakthroughs and a life of research, she remains blacklisted today. Her most infamous case involved New England Patriots star Aaron Hernandez, a convicted murderer who committed suicide at the age of twenty-seven—when he hanged himself with a bedsheet in prison—who had suffered with Stage 3 CTE.

There are four stages of CTE with Stage 4 being the most advanced. Stage 1 symptoms include headaches and a loss of attention and concentration. Stage 2 sees sufferers struggling with depression, mood swings and memory loss, as well as Stage 1 symptoms. There's also a greater risk of suicide at Stage 2. Stage 3 is all of the above and they are likely cognitively impaired by this point, with outbursts of aggression and impulsivity, too. Stage 4 victims have 'executive dysfunction', meaning there are cognitive, emotional, and behavioral problems. They have short-term memory loss, a form of dementia, along with balance issues, paranoia, and all of the symptoms from the previous stages. The damage to Hernandez's brain was so severe that in the 468 brains they'd used for research, they hadn't seen any as bad as Hernandez's, with the exception of some that had belonged to elderly patients. It would be speculation to link his CTE with the murder he was convicted of and the double murder he was acquitted of, and it's something McKee has steered clear of saying.

Despite being ostracized by the NFL, McKee retains clout all over the world. In 2017 she was voted Bostonian of the Year by the *Boston Globe*. In 2018 she was featured in *Time* as one of the hundred most influential people on the planet, alongside politicians, world leaders, and heads of industry. In the same year, the Alzheimer's Association awarded her with the Henry Wisniewski Lifetime Achievement Award. There's been a slew of other honors. She's gone on to find evidence of CTE in hundreds of athletes and has a stash of brains in an unmarked building on the VA premises. Inside there are twelve freezers, all kept at −80 degrees with between eighty and a hundred brains in each. Initial work is carried out in the bank and then, in a lab elsewhere on-site, brains are sliced thinly onto slides and dyed before being examined for diseases.

So far McKee has checked more than twenty-five boxers' brains. There are far more from football, at all levels, but McKee has yet to see one that has not had CTE from fighting. She remains a football fan but does so cautiously. "I happen to think it's a great sport but it's full of risk and dangers to the players and I can't watch it like I used to," she admitted. "I've never liked boxing. It's a tragic sport. Football is too. I've come to accept that. When you see twenty-year-olds with disease, there's no denying that CTE exists. I know there are many, many sports leagues and people that are very vocal about their criticism of my work, but there's no question in my mind that CTE is real. It's easily defined and it certainly affects football players—a high percentage of professional players but also a very disturbing number of amateur players. I've done twelve years of it and seen hundreds and hundreds of cases but it [seeing CTE] always stops me in my tracks, especially if it's a younger person where their life is cut short. It's very difficult to see, and it's very difficult to see that the world is still not acting on this and we're not solving the problem. We're just ignoring it."

While the NFL initially attempted to refute McKee's science, boxing has done nothing with it. There's been no detailed education with trainers, through commissions or sanctioning bodies, and no memos have gone out since CTE was confirmed. Nothing changed, yet this—punch-drunk syndrome—was boxing's problem before it was anyone else's.

McKee examined the brain of the late Scott LeDoux, who had tau in his motor neurons and in his spinal cord. There was also Greg Page, the veteran heavyweight who had been left paralyzed after a 2001 fight with Dale Crowe. Page slid out of his bed in 2009 and died of positional asphyxia, which is when your body position doesn't allow you to breathe. He was fifty years old. McKee also inspected the brain of Rulon "Curtis" Hatch, a forty-year-old former Canadian amateur and a three-time national champion. He had a history of paranoia and violence, his memory had started to play tricks on him, and he shot himself in his chest in front of his family on New Year's Eve in 2010. There was CTE in all three brains.

Many families still request anonymity for relatives who donate their brains. They just want their own answers while possibly helping to prevent a wider epidemic. And while McKee now has a plentiful and regular supply of brains, she needs more from a cross-section of athletes and fighters, particularly boxers who seem to be doing well despite exposure to trauma and those who appear to have been more resilient.

She also remains passionate about her work despite the high-level backlashes, criticism, and jealousy. She's not only on the front line working with the donated brains and spinal cords, but she tries to help those who have been affected by a loss. She's become close to many widows, brothers, sisters, and parents through the grieving process.

In many ways McKee has become the face of CTE. She sees it every day at work. She sees it in boxing. "[Boxing is] a huge risk and I don't like to see kids doing it," she added. But there are still plenty who disagree with her. Some think the work of J.A.N. Corsellis back in the 1970s is still the go-to work in neuropathology in relation to trauma.

"Corsellis was iconic of his time, but what I find perplexing is they [some colleagues around the world today] look at the Corsellis study as the end-all and be-all of CTE, and it was a study that was done in 1973 with medical techniques, staining techniques, that were available at the time, and there have been huge advances with specificity of staining. Also I think boxing has evolved over the past fifty years," McKee explained. "It's not quite the same sport of the '50s and '60s. There are different rules of engagement, different things, that just stands to reason. Although it's a hallmark paper, I don't think there's such a thing as classic CTE, which is what they want to call that Corsellis paper and then my work, which is modern CTE. That's just an attempt to try to marginalize my work, and the CTE that we see in boxers looks very similar to the CTE we see in football players, although by and large it tends to be more severe."

There is still work to do. CTE remains incurable and only detectable at autopsy when the tau protein can be seen under a microscope. "We need to diagnose it during life. That's probably the number one thing,"

McKee continued. "Then we can pull people out if they're still playing or if they're boxing and we have a better chance of treating it. There are lots of anti-tau drugs that are possible, anti-senso-nucleotides, there are vaccines even possible, and so if we were able to diagnose it early and follow it with a test, I think that would be the greatest step forward. We are looking at CSF [cerebrospinal fluid] spinal taps, we're looking at blood and plasma, we're looking at PET scans [positron emission tomography, which identifies diseases using radioactive tracers], but none of them are really very specific yet. My guess, and it is a guess, is five to ten years to be able to do it on an individual basis."

And that leads into one of the great head-scratchers facing scientists: Everyone is built differently. "There's definitely a genetic component to the risk," she continued. "Two people given the same exact exposure may have very different outcomes. One may be more susceptible, one may be more resistant, and probably one of the big factors is genetics. There are changes in some inflammatory pathways that are protected, that actually prevent CTE from getting severe, and there are probably also genes that make it more severe. [The gene] APO E4 makes it more severe. It doesn't increase your risk for it, but if you get it it's a more severe form and I'm sure that's just the tip of the iceberg."

And what of those who might have a predisposition to neurological illnesses, those who may have suffered with Alzheimer's, Parkinson's, or dementia later in life regardless of trauma? "What we see in older people with CTE, in their sixties, seventies, and on, is increased risk of other neurodegenerative diseases," McKee stated. "Once you get a neurodegenerative disease, your likelihood of developing a second one is much higher, and that seems to be a product of age, so depending on the age of those people they [retired fighters] could have had CTE plus AD [Alzheimer's], they could have had CTE plus Parkinson's, CTE plus ALS. We also know that CTE per se, pure CTE without any other neurodegenerative disease, can look just like Alzheimer's disease and be misdiagnosed as Alzheimer's disease. We also know it can look just like Parkinson's, so you don't have to have Parkinson's disease to have Parkinsonism or Parkinsonian symptoms. Sometimes it's just pure and simple CTE. But we also see the combo. And in ALS we have seen about 6 percent of people with CTE have a motor neuron disease with tau in their motor neurons, and we think they're etiologically [causally] related. Some people box and they're doing fine. Some people have what we call resilience or cognitive reserve. They do well until they don't do well, and then it's a pretty precipitous decline."

Then there are the behavioral traits of CTE. McKee contends that impulsivity, poor judgment, and aggression can make boxers better fighters and that because many boxers come from backgrounds of extreme poverty or trauma or both, it is hard to tell if some are destined to suffer with those behaviors.

McKee still faces considerable opposition but her many awards reaffirm her beliefs. They don't just represent her work; they represent her journey, of being marginalized, blacklisted, of battling the odds in gender wars—hidden or otherwise—often as the only woman in a room of alpha males. It's not an insignificant pleasure she derives from her spoils; it's not an ego driver. The awards serve to confirm that she's doing something right. That she's helping.

"That's exactly how I view the accolades," she said. "It's very validating. If my doctor peers can honor me for this work, I must be doing something right. There are still pockets of naysayers, and it's been an interesting field because it's been so widely in the public and none of my work was prior to this and I am not naturally a person who seeks attention—probably the opposite. But I've become this public figure, and that's been a very strange thing for me. What I've also found is it's not just big business and the people who hold the finances that control the science, they do, the money in science in general, the way they fund grants that support their point of view is clearly evident. Just like Coca-Cola supports work that shows sugar isn't a problem, major sports leagues support research that minimizes the effects of football or ice hockey. But the other thing that's been interesting is the scientists, and the absolute heat that I've received from other scientists. It's a hostility that I never thought would have existed, and I don't know their reasons but I think it has to do with attention. They don't like it that this work is getting so much attention, which is sad."

*　*　*

Yet McKee also has friends. One is Robert Cantu, one of the world's foremost neurosurgeons. In the early 1980s, Cantu had been a high school football coach at a time when the links between American football and head trauma had not been authoritatively made. Today, he works at Emerson Hospital in Concord, Massachusetts, and is a consultant to numerous NFL, NHL, and NBA teams. He's written hundreds of scientific publications, authored more than thirty books covering neurology and sports medicine—including *Boxing and Medicine*, which was published in 1995—and he is the go-to person for many when it comes to sports and concussion. His most recent book, entitled *Concussion and Our Kids*, looks at the safety aspects of children playing tackle football. On the walls of his office are signed pictures of NFL, NHL, and NBA stars, one of Nowinski in his wrestling attire and ones of boxers including former world super-welterweight champion Austin Trout and legendary warrior "Irish" Micky Ward.

His client list is extensive. He met Nowinski as a patient first—with Nowinski suffering from post-concussion syndrome as a lasting reminder of his wrestling days—but when Nowinski formed the Sports Legacy Institute, now known as the Concussion Legacy Foundation, they became colleagues.

Through his studies, whether they are football or boxing related, he believes exposure to and volume of trauma is the difference maker. Cantu cites the work of Kevin Bieniek at the University of Texas, whose studies have shown that if football players keep playing beyond high school they have a statistically greater chance of CTE, as much as five times higher. "It's clearly a volume relationship, and that is probably true with fighters as well," said Cantu. "It would be expected."

In terms of volume, this would include not just how many contests fighters have, but how often they spar and when they hang their gloves up. Cantu added: "Say five thousand [blows to the head] is that magic number and one boxer over a ten-round fight—I'm making this up—but say someone takes five hundred and the next guy takes two thousand because of the style. Well the guy who takes two thousand blows probably isn't going to fight as long as the guy who took five hundred to have the same cumulative effect."

There is no realistic way of keeping tabs on how many times someone has been hit, but for Cantu the solution is simple—reduce exposure. "Absolutely boxing can easily change that," insisted Cantu, who is now a senior advisor to the NFL Head, Neck, and Spine Committee, which was formerly the discredited NFL Concussion Committee. "Football players, at the National Football League level, where they've got agents and law-yers, they have been able to put through a bargaining agreement that says you can tackle each other only fourteen times during eighteen weeks of the season once the season starts, exclusive of game day; so practice, no tackling except less than once a week during the season, no tackling at all in the off-season. None. Zero. Zip. Because you want to reduce your chances for cumulative effect of head injury. Well, sure, boxers should not be sparring frequently; they should be doing a lot of conditioning work, resistive work, cardiovascular work, and punch work should mostly be on the mitts, on the bags, on other things if you're going to get creative. And some fighters are staying away from sparring except right before a fight but they're staying in shape year-round and working out year-round, just not taking blows to the head."

Only a few fighters actually do this. A change of culture is much needed in the sport, along with a change in thinking and education. Second-impact syndrome, when someone suffers a second concussion while still suffering from the first, is not widely discussed in boxing when it should be a regular part of the conversation.

The NFL has altered its return-to-play policies so when a player is hurt, they must be assessed. The player could be benched, withdrawn, or sent to the hospital, and symptoms must be monitored over time before any return—even to training—is permitted. In boxing, fighters will spar until a few days before a fight and then box. Or they may be back in the gym sparring a few days later. They often aren't examined and they certainly aren't monitored. Second-impact syndrome is one of the most serious threats to brain injury, both in the long and short term. In second-impact syndrome, the first hard hit has done more damage than anyone suspects and then the boxer takes a follow-up shot and life can be irreparably changed. A fighter can be hurt in sparring and still not be healed by fight night, when disaster can strike.

"If you're symptomatic that week, if the symptoms persist, then you're at risk of second-impact," Cantu said. "And that's very import-ant because that should be a reason to stop the fight. We all know why fights don't get stopped, but you can get second-impact within the same fight. The guy who essentially can't remember anything from the third round on, he was at risk for second-impact. Whether he got it or not is another issue. Second-impact syndrome, we can also call it dysregulation syndrome, meaning that there is a disruption of normal blood flow to the brain so there's swelling of the brain, by that I mean vascular congestion in the brain. It's not swelling like edema, like fluid in the interstitial spaces between cells, but congestion of blood in the brain. Second-impact syndrome is that—it's vascular congestion and it's dis-autoregulation. I don't know of a boxer who was killed by a single blow. I only know of boxers who were killed by an accumulation of blows. If they had a subdural, in many cases it could be removed, but the brains went on to malignant swelling, which is the vascular congestion that killed them. And the best example of that would be Duk Koo Kim . . . who took tremendous punishment [in his fight with Ray Mancini] and collapsed at the end of the fight. Within an hour the neurosurgeon had him in the operating room and the blood clot out, but the brain just swelled up and he died. . . . I've seen malignant brain swelling when there's been a subdural with a single blow, yes. Motorcyclists that hit trees, car accidents at tremendous speeds, . . . [but] I've never seen it from repetitive lower accelerations like you see in boxing. I believe it's the accumulation of blows over time that lead to this malicious increased risk of brain damage."

Through the years, Cantu has seen changes and patterns emerge. One dramatic alteration has been on his view of the cavum septum pellucidum. A gap could naturally be there, but generally fighters have a much wider space between the ventricles and that, he now believes, is unnatural. When fighters do hear from commissions that their brain scans have changed, it's usually because the gap has grown wider.

"We believe that the large cavums you're not born with, and the fenestrated [perforated] cavums, where you've got shearing of the wall that pulls apart, that's from trauma," he said. "That's not because you were born with it. So yes, a small cavum septum pellucidum that is perfectly formed, you don't know if it's congenital or not, unless it's getting bigger over time, so you follow it but a big cavum with fenestrations, you were not born that way."

Because boxing is a fragmented sport, some fighters may not have their first brain scans until after two-hundred amateur fights. They may already have a cavum septum pellucidum. They may have had one anyway, but, without a series of MRI scans, you can't tell and there's no progress to follow.

Cantu has been involved in boxing for years. He's worked with the USA Boxing amateur program, and at Boston University he's been involved with the Association of Ringside Physicians.

There's no clear answer about whether a dehydrated boxer is more at risk of developing CTE, but Cantu has investigated boxing and rehydration. This is a sport where fighters starve themselves, fast, and boil what's left of their minerals away in saunas before stepping onto the scales in a vastly depleted state. Some link that to brain damage, though it remains unproven at this stage.

"'Don't know' is the honest answer," conceded Cantu, who figures that the brain of a dehydrated boxer has more room 'to slosh around in the skull' and the risk is greater if there's a small brain in a large skull.

"So a dehydrated state would be bad," Cantu said. "Most of the boxers are hydrated up by the time they fight, but whether the brain's had enough time to be rehydrated is another question. The bloodstream can be rehydrated but whether each cell in the brain has expanded to its normal size, we don't really know."

And since Cantu first became involved in boxing several decades ago, the landscape has changed. There were few women in boxing then; now women can steal the show and top the bills. Are they at equal risk? Again, that is unknown, partly because there aren't enough brains in the brain bank to study.

"We know that women statistically get more concussions in sports that both men and women play . . . but concussions don't correlate with CTE so we can't really use that data to say conclusively that women are more at risk from CTE," stated Dr. Cantu. "The reason I worry particularly about women is, generally speaking, their necks are not as strong, they're not as developed. They can make their necks stronger with the same exercises guys do, but they'll never be as strong as guys because of the lack of testosterone levels that not only make your muscles stronger but make your muscles bigger and bulkier. And your neck is a shock absorber for a punch to the extent that it's like the HANS device is to automobile racing. . . . In the HANS device, when you can completely affix your neck to the back of your driver's seat so it can't move independently of the driver's seat, you don't see concussions. . . . We've seen in NASCAR—since the HANS device has been mandated—that concussions have virtually been eliminated. They occasionally occur but they're very, very uncommon. That is also why in boxing the most dangerous state by far is when the boxer's hurt, so that natural avoidance of a punch, seeing a punch coming and so tensing your muscles to take a punch is gone, and that relaxed, groggy state is awful for boxers."

Other sports have looked at cutting-edge safety improvements, whether it's motor racing and the HANS device or football with helmets, but there is not much that can be done to make boxing safer. Fighters have hand wraps, mouthpieces, and gloves. The size of the gloves have been tinkered with over the years in an attempt to improve safety. The amateur code has largely lost headgear, and they're only used by professionals for sparring. But they do not protect the brain, and Cantu is well-placed to discuss them, having reviewed football helmets in medical papers over the years.

"Let's talk about what isn't debatable," he began. "Headgear for fighters protects against cuts, protects against broken noses, protects against eye injury, so from that alone it's appropriate—in my opinion—for amateur boxers, certainly when they're sparring, and I believe when they're fighting. There have been studies that I think are very poorly done that have suggested that boxers wearing headgear think they're safer and therefore drop their hands in clinches, take more blows, and wind up having more concussions. And this is [the International Boxing Association's] work. Most of us don't think they were really well-done studies, and we do think headgear is protective. Does it protect against concussion? Obviously not. Does it protect against getting CTE? Obviously not. Does it give you some protection attenuating blows to the head? Yes. So, I think for the reasons of it protecting what you know it does—the face, the eyes, the cuts—that alone is reason to wear headgear. The marginal protection it gives you beyond that, for the brain, is probably the concept lesser is always better. So it's not protecting in any big way, but it's giving you some protection and I would suggest it is worn. Now the arguments against it, that boxers feel more emboldened because they've got head protection is wrong—it's education—that they shouldn't be thinking that way. The other argument is the headgear allows the glove a rough surface to hit and can therefore more forcefully whip the head than if you had something slick that your gloves would bounce off, which you're not going to see, because history's history. But you can make the argument that the boxer's helmet on the outside should look more like other athletic helmets so that the boxer's blow will slide off easier."

Of course, it's not just what fighters do in the arena and in the gym that affects them, but how they live away from the sport. With brain injuries a risk, adding a concoction of drugs and alcohol—when mood swings, impulsivity, and depression are already at play—is a potential disaster zone. Cantu says it's not a good mix and can either make matters worse or mask symptoms or make them appear worse than they are. But fighters have battled addictions for decades, whether it was John L. Sullivan or Gene Tunney's drinking, someone's gambling, Johnny Tapia's coke snorting, or Mike Tyson's marijuana smoking, whatever it may be, fighters often have addictive personalities.

Then there are those who took their own lives. The list of boxing suicides is painfully long and stems back further than Frenchman Fred Bretonnel, who hung himself at the age of twenty-three in 1928. It includes Jock McAvoy, Billy and Ernie Smith, Edwin Valero, Ricky Womack, Darren Sutherland, Alexis Arguello, Billy Papke, Kid McCoy, Tarmo Uusivirta, and Billy Ward. There are many more, but most of these men had either battled depression, made bad life decisions, or their lives had begun to spiral irreversibly out of control.

"That's a segue into an issue that needs to be studied tremendously, the whole suicide issue," Cantu went on. "How much is CTE contributing? How much are addictive behaviors contributing? How much [are alcohol] and drugs contributing? How much is genetics contributing? Because some of these people have family histories of depression, anxiety, and so on. There are a number of people who are doing research in that area right now that I hope one day will give us the answers. There are people saying today they have the answers; I don't believe them. I don't think we do. It's a mix, but I don't know how much is contributing to what."

There is a chance that some may have been destined to struggle neurologically in life, or they may have genetically been at a greater risk before they started boxing. Cantu doesn't think it's as straightforward as those with the APO E4 gene being more vulnerable, despite that being the gene that's involved in Alzheimer's. There have been tests that show that those who have APO E4 might have a predisposition; and so if they have a higher exposure to trauma then they could be more likely to suffer from cognitive or behavioral problems. He is certain that there are genetic combinations at play. Some fighters can sustain concussions easily, but others, like Muhammad Ali, for example, was almost impossible to knock down or knock out so he could take more blows, which only means he got punched more often.

CTE is a highly serious issue itself, but it could also be an accelerant to other neurological illnesses, something Cantu is almost certain of. Of the great fighters who died and were diagnosed with dementia, Parkinson's, ALS, or Alzheimer's over the years, there is not only a chance that it was just CTE misdiagnosed, but it could have triggered different medical problems.

"You got dementia, Alzheimer's, Parkinson's but you got it twenty or thirty years earlier," Cantu said. "Absolutely. For those people who are going to be mixed CTE and Alzheimer's, CTE and Parkinson's, CTE and frontotemporal dementia, I think you're right on and I think that's the way most of us are thinking. But there are pure cases of CTE, and in those cases they're probably not an accelerant, just the result. [Those cases of old boxers] could be CTE or CTE plus one of the others, but CTE for sure. The ALS that we're seeing with CTE, the brains look like CTE, the spinal cord looks like ALS. So we're seeing CTE with ALS, about 10 percent of the CTE brains have had ALS."

Inherently the talk of fighters knowing what they sign up for relates to the night of a contest, the chance of cuts and bruises, the heartache, the danger of being injured on the big stage—it's not years from when they first pull on gloves, or years after they've taken them off for the last time. Cantu contends that fighters will ignore the possibilities and the dangers and just think, 'It's not going to happen to me.' He's making it his mission to put forward the most accurate risk-reward data he can, but, other than that, it's up to adults to pursue whatever legal path society allows them to.

"The problem I have with [kids boxing] is they don't understand, they're really not informed," he explained. "They're almost never fully using informed consent. And youngsters are more vulnerable, so I would say boxing, for youths, should be without head blows if you're going to do it, but you can't convince anybody to do that."

You certainly can't monitor it, either. But Cantu is determined to keep moving forward, to provide information and then let fighters make up their minds even though he concedes more knowledge is needed across the board, even at Boston University, even in his office.

Cantu continued: "[Boxers] don't have the protection and the awareness that NFL players have with their pension plans and everything else, to the extent that the plight and the risk and the rewards can be made more known. I hope it leads to governing bodies doing the right thing, which is not to eliminate it but to regulate it in a safer way. . . . [T]here are many more activities that are more dangerous than boxing that society doesn't say you can't do, so I'm pretty sure it's not going to stop boxing or it would have been done a long time ago."

* * *

While McKee is not a fight fan and Cantu has tried to help the sport, Chris Nowinski is nonplussed, even more so because of his journey through concussion, trauma, and damage. Nowinski is the brain collector in Boston. He gets the subjects and delivers the organs to McKee. He's also a passionate advocate of keeping children safe in contact sports, and that means reducing if not removing head trauma from games at the youth level and under. His 2006 book, *Head Games*, looks at American football and kids. As a former athlete, he's also protecting the stars, although he realizes that boxing is different. Fighters are on their own. After Liverpool's former cruiserweight champion Tony Bellew was knocked out by Oleksandr Usyk in Manchester in 2018, the Englishman was allowed to give post-fight interviews in the ring. He repeated himself over and over, a sure sign of concussion and head injury. He also said he didn't know in what round the fight was finished or what punches brought about his downfall, yet he was in the ring for several minutes talking to radio and TV broadcasters.

"If you compare boxing to what's happening in football or other sports, there's virtually no one looking out for the athletes," Nowinski said. "The NFL has a policy that if you have a concussion, you're not ever exposed to the media just in case you say or do something you wouldn't have done without a brain issue. So the idea that someone was being interviewed after being knocked out and that's normal, and that the announcers were okay with that, television was okay with that, it means there's no scrutiny and there's no one looking out for the boxers."

The red flags that were ignored by the British Boxing Board of Control and promoters—anyone in the chain of command that could have stopped the news outlets from getting their pound of flesh from a broken but still generous man—are rife throughout the sport today. Yet it's boxers who are most at risk; it is, after all, boxing's problem.

"If boxing has problems it's because we know CTE and concussions are a bigger problem in boxing than any other sport but that information is not being utilized," Nowinski admitted. "CTE was first identified in boxers. If you go and watch *Requiem for a Heavyweight*, if you go and watch *On the Waterfront* with Marlon Brando playing a punch-drunk boxer, it was known in the 1950s and earlier that boxers get punch-drunk. Then, as boxing lost the cachet, it appeared that there's no incentive to keep on talking about it in the boxing community."

Nowinski's Concussion Legacy Foundation, with a small staff, doesn't work in boxing. Their priority is football and keeping millions safe. That boxing is a high-risk pursuit should be well-known enough, even if the long-term dangers are not. "The assumption is that people already know [that boxing is dangerous], there doesn't need to be any additional work done on this, and there's very few children still doing it in America; so we focus on sports that drive the national conversation and we are here to protect kids," Nowinski said. "No one pays attention to boxing and if anyone talks about taking it away from kids the argument is that it's their best alternative; because wherever those kids are boxing it's keeping them off the streets, it's giving them father figures, it becomes a socioeconomic and race discussion rather than a health discussion."

Yet with the research at his disposal, Nowinski insists that children at age eleven or under should not be getting punched in the head. "You shouldn't be allowed to hit kids in the head while their brain's still developing and they can't understand the risks they're being exposed to," he said. "They shouldn't be boxing with head blows probably until about eighteen because the science is so clear, but we primarily focus on age fourteen for team sports, partially because most kids aren't playing those sports beyond age eighteen anyway and we don't have the evidence to say a four-year career in the sport is going to put you at huge risk. But no, kids should not be boxing at eleven."

That's the current start age for children in most countries, but the gyms are unsupervised. Children are taught to box and fight younger than age eleven. It's the sloppy setup of boxing, with no one umbrella organization, that creates a barrier that prevents people like Nowinski from trying to help. He's worked with the NBA, the NFL, the NHL, and the WWE, among others. In boxing, where would he even begin? Nevada? New York? New Jersey? Texas? The United Kingdom? Germany? The WBC? The IBF?

"There's no one person to talk to and that also matters," he agreed. "When we're talking about kids and soccer in America, we focus our conversation on US Soccer. With boxing, there's no way to organize national change, and we're a small organization with ten people and we have to spend our time where we can make the most difference for the most people, and [with] boxing, I don't know if there's a path forward to changing it. Nobody seems to care within boxing. That's the issue."

Yet it's not just that. Yes, lack of structure is a significant obstacle, but head trauma has been written into more-than-century-old laws, and for Nowinski that is just wrong. "It's so absurd that you factor concussions into the sport with eight counts, you're accepting concussions as part of it," he explained, while suggesting a three-count would be better. "Concussion is part of boxing. The recovery from concussion is institutionalized into the count. If you knock someone down with a punch and they don't pop right back up, they have a concussion. If you give them time to get their bearings and stand up, now you're letting them box while clearly concussed. And that's the rules. So if you actually cared about concussions in what you were doing, there would no longer be a count; you would just say you don't get ten seconds. If you're not up in three seconds or even immediately, you're done, unless it's a punch to the stomach. But the idea that somebody gets punched in the head and they get ten seconds to recover is unethical."

It's why Nowinski has been so outspoken about the return-to-play policies in football, not just the dangers of second-impact syndrome but the potential long-term harm of getting hurt again too soon after a first hard hit.

The education for football players and other athletes has filtered down from the top. Without a centralized organization, there's nowhere for boxers to get educated, no go-to source, no self-help manuals, and no union. NFL stars now get help from the NFL Players Association and they have annual training explaining what concussion is. In boxing, Nowinski wouldn't even know where to start the education process.

"In theory, it would be great to create a scared-straight video where you can say, 'This is actually what's happening to your brain when you do this' and force people to watch it," he reckoned. "I don't know how to enforce that."

The best way to spread the word would be through gyms and trainers. That seems incredibly unlikely. Most trainers are enigmas; many of them are old-school and too many of them don't understand the long-term risks when they should be the most informed.

The Concussion Legacy Foundation has had breakthroughs in MMA, working alongside Rose Gracie from the Gracie family with a Gracie Concussion Challenge. Fighters are being taught about the threat of competing while concussed, carrying a head injury and going into a fight when already damaged, even mildly. Many Gracies from the historic Brazilian jiu-jitsu line have pledged to donate their brains, to learn more about CTE, and to educate their trainers so they can pass their knowledge down.

Meanwhile, Nowinski still sees one of the main problems boxing has is with fighters thinking nothing bad will happen to them. The strategy of the Concussion Legacy Foundation is to educate about the risks of damage through the global media. Athletes making their brain pledges public also helps raise awareness, and the WWE has supported the Foundation and funds some of the work it does. "I do annual training for the wrestlers, and the referees know what we're learning about concussions and CTE and they've embraced all that work to try to make it safer," Nowinski said. "Whether they just want to do it to keep the guys and girls healthy so they can stay on the road year-round, at least they're listening. Because you can wrestle forever. You can wrestle for thirty years if you take care of yourself. It's not like you can replace John Cena tomorrow with the next superstar. So the wrestlers are informed of the risks and they control the risks. It's not boxing where you have to get hit in the head. At the beginning some people thought I went soft because they didn't understand. Now all wrestlers treat me like gold because part of the reason they're wrestlers and not boxers is because they want to have the excitement of it but without really getting hurt. The whole goal is to not get hurt, so they're an enlightened group. If they find out they're doing something that's getting them hurt, they'll stop."

Many pro wrestlers have died young. When death rates are tracked in sports, boxing is not often highly ranked, but it's the long, slow deaths that nobody's tracking.

"You forget how to eat," Nowinski said of the final stages of CTE. "You forget how to swallow. Saliva gets into your lungs and you choke to death. Pneumonia, risk-taking behavior, depression, your ability to exercise [and] take care of yourself, and less direct things that affect your life. I've [also] just seen enough people kill themselves or others, who were once great guys that you sort of assume there might be a connection there [with murder and suicide]. Last week there was a Harvard football player who was thirty years old who killed his mother and was then killed by the police."

For Nowinski, the goal is spreading the word of CTE and sharing knowledge to try to minimize its place in society. "The vision is we talk about a world without CTE, so that means to prevent it in the short term and eventually maybe we're treating it. . . . [O]ur mission statement is concussion safety without compromise, meaning that we're doing everything we can to prevent as many as we can and then if they're happening, identify and treat them as best we can," added Nowinski. "So in sports there'd be no purposeful head contact until a certain age. Right now it's fourteen, it might be different later. Science changes. But you're not heading soccer balls, you're not getting punched in the head, you're not tackling people, all of those things are terrible ideas for children's brains. And then with the adults we're trying to minimize risk. So it would be no sparring, no tackling in your NFL practices. You just limit exposure when it's not for the money and then when it's for the money you have the rules that are ethical."

Nowinski is a campaigner. He's hugely knowledgeable, incredibly driven, and ambitious. He doesn't just have plans that will change the sporting landscape; he's motivated by protecting kids. For a while, the motivation was to tackle the NFL; the football giants were lying in their defense of their sport. Then, once the tables turned on the NFL and they paid out millions upon millions, including a million-dollar donation to Boston University and the Concussion Legacy Foundation for their research, Nowinski just wanted to see fewer people succumb to the brain diseases he has seen impair, cripple, and eventually kill friends of his from the football and wrestling worlds.

It was only when he'd taken on his own damage that he started to learn. "How am I, an Ivy League graduate, that when I got kicked in the head and blacked out I carried on," he recalled of the night his life changed in wrestling against one of the Dudley Boys in the WWE.

"If you care about your brain health you shouldn't be boxing. In some sports you can say you don't know the risks, but with boxing you know that getting punched in the head is bad. In football you can say, 'I'm going to tackle safely' or whatever. In boxing you might think 'I'm not going to let them punch me,' but eventually that stops."

Yet the stigma remains. There seems to be sadness for fallen NFL giants and gridiron greats but boxers are "punchy"? "There was no sympathy and no understanding of it, so wives would often protect their husbands, not let them go out, not let people see them and their decline," Nowinski said of old fighters. "They would not get support and . . . [they'd] become isolated because there was no appreciation of what was happening. In the U.S. we've completely changed the concussion culture; that's spreading globally. We've started to change the future of CTE because we're starting to change how we play the sports and when kids start playing contact. There's no headers [in soccer] before eleven and within ten years that will be a global phenomenon."

✱ ✱ ✱

So, although there is progress elsewhere, boxing is a long way behind the curve, whether it is in comparison to professional wrestling, mixed martial arts, or football. Fighters are still getting damaged, families are still covering it up, and no one's talking about it—not often enough and not loudly enough.

Throughout the founding years of the Concussion Legacy Foundation, Floyd Mayweather ruled the boxing world and possibly became the first billion-dollar athlete, earning hundreds of millions a night for several fights. He was a master craftsman, specializing in hitting and not getting hit, but his trainer and uncle, Roger, was struggling toward the end. Roger had been a two-time world champion, a huge puncher who was badly knocked out a handful of times in his defeats. In 2014, Roger was interviewed on a YouTube channel about the long-term effects of boxing and whether he was concerned about his future. "Anytime somebody fights a hundred times, fifty times, seventy . . . something is going to happen," he replied. "You don't know. I don't know. I look at Ali, I could see the changes from him. . . . Somebody says the way you talk, the way you do this, the way you do that. I don't think about it, but when they see me, they know. Yeah, that many fights, you've got to be punchy. . . . The grind is taking a beating over time; over time is what messed the fighter up. That's why Muhammad Ali's messed up. . . . I miss boxing. I liked boxing. Do I have injuries from boxing? I really don't know. . . . But I can look back and say to myself, I think that I did what I wanted to do in boxing and, sure, something [is] going to happen one way or the other. . . . One way or another something's going to happen. And that's what happened to me, something happened."

He'd had seventy-two pro fights, winning fifty-nine and losing thirteen with six by stoppage and Roger started to go downhill rapidly.

"My uncle, Roger Mayweather, has lost a lot of memory from the sport of boxing," Floyd told fighthype.com. "And it's sad that he's only in his fifties but it seems as if he's an old man that's in his eighties, from the sport of boxing. Boxing is wear and tear on the body."

Floyd said his uncle had suffered with mood swings, he'd forgotten combinations on the pads, he didn't know who his nephew was anymore, and was wandering off and getting lost. He was working on getting him help. He needed a caretaker.

"Roger, he's not doing good," said his brother, Floyd Sr., in 2018, adding that Roger was losing his sight, his independence, and that he was depressed. Away from the public eye, Roger would deteriorate, a casualty of war.

And still the cycle continued.

"Adonis Stevenson is playing out as we speak," Steve Farhood said of the injured former WBC light-heavyweight champion, who suffered a severe brain injury in 2018 in a fight with Oleksandr Gvozdyk. "I spoke to Adonis and he's doing very well, much better than was anticipated, but it really bothers me that in cases where there aren't fatalities, where a fighter suffers long-term effects, that we tend to forget them. We tend to ignore them. If a fighter suffers a subdural hematoma and makes it, obviously the most dramatic example is Gerald McClellan, but if a fighter makes it then for two weeks, or a month, six or eight weeks, everybody is concerned, wishes for the best, and then they're forgotten. That's a terrible thing. Gerald McClellan should never be forgotten, and hopefully Adonis Stevenson—while he looks like he might be doing very well—hopefully he will never be forgotten. But that's a very upsetting thing to me because these are not disposable athletes, these are not disposable commodities. It's grossly unfair. Life goes on for boxing, but that life stops for the fighters and they're thrown from the back of the treadmill."

8
The Study

A QUEST FOR ANSWERS

While work is being done in Boston to find answers from the dead, across the United States in Las Vegas, research is being undertaken to get answers from the living.

Inside the Lou Ruvo Center's Cleveland Clinic a little north of the Strip, Dr. Charles Bernick leads the Professional Fighters Brain Health Study (PFBHS), working with hundreds of boxers and mixed martial artists to track brain health and symptoms. There's a whole range of athletes who are signed up, from young amateurs to retired legends and Dr. Bernick is collecting data to determine, among other things, whether careers in boxing and mixed martial arts (MMA) play a role in fighters contracting Alzheimer's, Parkinson's, ALS, and other neurological or dementia-related illnesses. Bernick is also trying to find biomarkers (medical signs) that can show fighters whether they are at a greater risk of being affected by CTE in their lives, either during their career or after the final bell.

Bernick's fighter study has four main goals:

(1) Detect the earliest and most subtle signs of brain injury in those exposed to head trauma using MRI and other clinical measures.

(2) Determine what risk factors make an individual exposed to head trauma more likely to develop chronic neurological disorders.

(3) Identify those individuals, by tracking brain function over a period of time, who are progressing toward developing long-term neurological diseases such as CTE, Alzheimer's, or Parkinson's.

(4) Provide information to guide athletes and empower them to make informed decisions.

The study differs from others in the field because it monitors the long-term rather than the short-term effects of concussion and head trauma. Fighters who want to participate are tested for free. If they live in the United States, their expenses are covered. Assessments include a look at their brain health and function, MRI scans, exams of their cognitive abilities, speech tests, and blood sampling (for genetic and protein testing). In addition, participants fill out questionnaires about their moods, sleep, impulsivity, and they take a neurological balance test.

More than eight hundred fighters have signed up for the study, which started in 2011 and involves annual tests. It is an open-ended project that could last more than a decade and should give scientists a more holistic view of repetitive head trauma. Already, researchers have made several significant findings. For example, they have been able to see changes in certain areas of a fighters' brain using MRI. Scientists have also been able to track changes that show a correlation between greater exposure to head trauma and a decline in performance on tests of processing speed in active fighters.

By tallying each athlete's "fight exposure score," which uses age, number of fights, and fights per year, researchers can also now provide rough estimates of a fighter's risk of performing poorly on certain cognitive tests. Crucially, scientists have found both boxers and MMA fighters may have markers of long-term brain injury in their blood. It will take more time, money, and work, but those working on the project are trying to understand how much fighting is too much.

Bernick has become one of the go-to guys in the quest for knowledge about fighters and their brains. Having earned his medical degree from the University of Texas Southwestern Medical School, he specialized in

Alzheimer's, dementia, and memory loss. He joined the Lou Ruvo Center in 2009 when it opened. In 2011, he was the first neurologist assigned to track brain damage over time in fighters. He understands the risks of the sport but hopes that through testing, the risks can be reduced. Bernick also presents seminars about the study worldwide.

"[I think] what we really need to understand is—for two people who have had relative exposure—why somebody comes out well and another one doesn't," Bernick explained. "There's the obvious things—somebody just gets hit more or their style of fighting, the way they train, that adds to a cumulative exposure issue. But we're exploring different variables. Some people have ways to clear and repair injuries better than others, and if we can find and discover those things, we can use them."

Bernick admits that many people view symptoms of head trauma in boxers as just how boxers end up. It's what happens. In American football, it kicked off a crisis. In boxing, it's seen as part of the culture. He contends that there's little understanding of the long-term risks even if the discussion in other sports has marginally crossed over in to boxing. "Because for so long it was thought it was just boxing and people just don't care," stated Bernick. "They really don't care."

Plenty of fighters and trainers believe that boxers are affected not just by the punches they have taken but by the combination of those blows along with drugs, alcohol, and a hard lifestyle away from the ring. Yet Bernick is not so quick to believe the two are linked. "Hard to know," he said. "We never know what's the chicken and what's the egg. Is it just people accumulate injury and then develop bad habits or is it the bad habits that compound it? [S]ome of the physical signs, the Parkinsonism, the speech, some of these motor signs . . . [would] be hard to explain by alcoholism or a lot of alcohol. It probably cuts both ways."

The study does not ask fighters to undergo drug tests. And it is not just drug and alcohol use that may have affected the fighters. It is their entire histories. When you consider the diseases some boxers have, are they hereditary? And when you consider personality changes, mood alterations, and depression, do they come from a sad upbringing, a broken relationship—or are their brains damaged?

"It's hard to know," Bernick continued. "We haven't analyzed people about their past or their personality. Did they have a morbid state? Were they poor learners in school and do they have attention deficit disorders?

Does depression or bipolar illness run in their family? . . . Is it the head trauma that's causing the bizarre behaviors? [Or] is it because that's their kind of personality to begin with? Did the boxing bring out or accentuate the person's premorbid [before disease onset] personality because of an injury or whatever? I think in some cases it's probably a little of each."

It's a methodical approach, to collate family history, school records and performance, and explore backgrounds to see what behavior might be attributed to trauma and what it actually part of their personality.

Then there are the links to other neurological illnesses, the type that Bernick has spent his professional life observing and treating. He's clearly fascinated trying to find the common threads between the degeneration he has witnessed and the fighting backgrounds of the study participants.

Bernick believes that everyone has a reserve that is reduced with head trauma. The more head trauma one receives, the more the well runs dry. The injuries to the brain cause cells and fibers to degenerate, and so those predisposed to Alzheimer's or Parkinson's may suffer with it earlier than they would have. CTE is different, however, in that it can only be caused by repetitive head trauma. What he wants to know is exactly how much is too much? What time limits should a fighter have on his career? Should there be a maximum number of rounds, fights, and training camps?

"Someone who fights once a year could maybe go until he's forty whereas maybe someone who fights three times a year may need to check out at thirty-two," said Bernick. "That's a goal of this study, too. If we had an imaging marker to determine whether you're starting to accumulate damage or even if there was some sort of battery of cognitive tests—which are actually available now, iPad-based tests that can be done—and if someone has a trajectory where they're declining on these tests at a certain rate then you [would] feel more confident to have [that person] stop their career. . . . Hopefully there are some biological measures that can assess each person individually and determine whether they should continue fighting or not. Using arbitrary cut-offs, I guess that's a start, but again we don't really have any science about that."

Then you have fighters who buck the trend. What about Bernard Hopkins, a light-heavyweight champion until the age of fifty? Or George Foreman, a world heavyweight champion in his mid-forties? What they did was inspirational, but it fostered a dangerous belief in aging fighters that if Hopkins and Foreman could do it, so could they. And there are plenty of other dangerous precedents in the sport, not least of which is its macho culture, which encourages fighters to lie about being hurt and to fight on regardless of their injuries.

Bernick says it is down to the trainers to keep fighters safe and that licensed coaches should be taught about concussion and head trauma protocols so they understand the long- and short-term effects. He appreciates it is not an easy conversation for a trainer to have but they can have a positive spin. Rather than say someone shouldn't spar or fight because they're hurt, they should be told that they shouldn't spar because it will hurt their performance and they would be at risk of getting a second concussion.

It's apparent that some fighters and trainers are aware of acute dangers, but they don't necessarily consider the long-term, chronic risks. They might not think it is because of boxing that a retired fighter who was in apparently good health a decade after hanging up the gloves suddenly experiences a drastic downturn. That is one of the things Bernick wants to learn: What prompts a fighter to be fine years after retiring and then suddenly decline? "It's hard to know," he said again. "It may not be related at all to them being a boxer or maybe it reduced their reserve and so the disease starts and it manifests itself much faster. So, again, we've got to learn more."

Bernick is especially hoping to develop a biological test or scan that can reveal the tau protein produced by CTE that gradually breaks down brain cells, causing the reduced state fighters find themselves in while they're still alive. Various testing measures being considered include tau imaging, blood tests, as well as looking at another element, called neurofilament lighting, which reflects injuries to the fibers in the brain. As things stand, scientists need to wait for an autopsy to discover the extent of someone's damage.

"We won't have the luxury of that in most people; but if we did, we could compare them and it would give us confidence to measure what's truly happening in the brain," Bernick added. "That's where the field is going, and all these things are quite feasible, they're just not ready for prime time just yet."

* * *

Bernick's study is being financed in part by some of America's promotional powerhouses and networks: Top Rank Boxing, Golden Boy Promotions,

Haymon Boxing, the UFC, Bellator, and Spike TV. For once, many of the different groups are on the same side.

"What was a pleasant surprise was the enthusiasm of the combat-sports industry, which of course was unlike what we had here in American football," Bernick said. "We had the support of our athletic commission [Nevada] right from the start. . . . I think the playing field is totally different [than in football]. In combat sports there are no unions and people are independent contractors so I don't know if the promoters had as much to worry about as far as their responsibility. On the other hand, I got the impression—at least in terms of the people that we've dealt with—that they're supportive. They want to make the sport safer as best as we can. No one's going to eliminate the sport, but are there ways to detect damage, to change training habits? There may be ways to impose procedures and policies that would help long-term brain safety."

Top Rank boss Bob Arum, whose wife Lovee serves on the board of directors at the Lou Ruvo Center, is one of the donating promoters. "Absolutely we've invested in it," said Arum. "With Dr. Bernick's special research on boxers and MMA fighters, they're doing a great job. And while you cannot eliminate it completely, you can, with monitoring as I understand it, really prevent the worst cases and stop that punch-drunk syndrome before it takes effect. You can do that with testing, and everybody involved in boxing, from the commissions to the promoters, want to see that done. We are all obviously concerned."

He thinks there is more awareness in young fighters than there was in the old days and believes boxing's protocols are already in line with other sports, citing the rule that if a fighter is knocked out, he is not allowed to box for ninety days. "When you're talking to active fighters . . . a lot of them are interested in their health and will say, 'I know people who are punch-drunk, I don't want to get that way.' Or they say, 'If I was going to get that way I would stop'," added Arum.

And unlike much in boxing, with different sanctioning and governing bodies either failing to work together or actively trying to usurp one another, Bernick and the Lou Ruvo Center have friends in the global health community, including the brain bank in Boston and universities in Washington and Sweden.

One person who speaks highly of Bernick is Dr. Robert Cantu. "I think his boxer study is hugely important and I think it's going to reinforce what we're already seeing at [Boston University]," Cantu said. "At least in my eyes, it takes a lot of repetitive brain trauma for most people to start to show cognitive behavioral or mood difficulties. Although we still don't know the risk definitively for CTE because we don't have that prospective study, [Bernick] will get as close as you can in boxers when he's done another ten, fifteen, or twenty years of his study."

* * *

Although he doesn't have firm guidelines in place for older boxers, based on his research and that of others Bernick believes head contact shouldn't be allowed before the age of fourteen. "The brain doesn't really completely form or stop its development until you're in your twenties, but certainly around twelve, thirteen, fourteen, there's a time when a lot of changes in the brain are occurring. So the earlier you start, it may predispose you to either greater deficits or maybe increase your likelihood of getting certain diseases," he said. "With our work, there did seem to be a slight difference in boxing younger as a group, that's what Boston University found, but we are looking at people who made it to professional level so we don't know if starting at eighteen . . . is that okay? My own sense if you want to err on safety is you don't start any of these impact sports or contact sports until you're about fourteen."

Yet sparring often happens with children far younger. It is not uncommon to see YouTube videos or social media posts of ten- and eleven-year-olds knocking each other woozy. Sparring to the head is allowed in most gyms around the world beginning at age eleven. And boxers at a young age are taught to disguise pain and to be like the tough guys they idolize on TV. Some of the top Mexican fighters, like Julio Cesar Chavez and Marco Antonio Barrera, turned professional at fifteen and were fighting grown men. Meanwhile, by the age of fourteen, Puerto Rican hero Wilfred Benitez had moved to New York, where he was boxing in the roughest gyms. He sparred wars with Hall of Famer and former world champion Emile Griffith and became a world champion at a record-breaking age of seventeen. By the time he was thirty-seven, he could no longer feed or clothe himself. In a 1997 *New York Times* article entitled "Too Many Beatings; The Boxer's Disease Haunts Wilfred Benitez and His Family," journalist Evelyn Nieves wrote, "The sport that had made him the youngest boxing champion in history at 17 was going to finish him off at 38." In 2018, at the age of fifty-nine, Benitez was flown to Chicago for emergency care. He'd lost two decades to darkness, dependent on family and friends.

Perhaps those early, halcyon and celebrated years learning his trade came at a great cost. Perhaps it's the reason why having lost just once in forty-five fights, Benitez was hammered by Tommy Hearns and lost seven of his next seventeen fights. He boxed until the age of thirty-two. Although his late mother, Clara, had noticed changes in him in 1986, he had four more fights in 1990, getting licensed in Phoenix, Tucson, Denver, and Winnipeg.

And as far as the old scientists saying that it was the come-forward sluggers, the journeymen or the sparring partners who were damaged the worst, Benitez was a boxing mastermind, called "The Radar" because it was believed he was hardly ever hit.

In fact, fighting styles are one of the ways Bernick's study assesses a fighter's exposure to punishment, but they don't have the answers on who's most at risk yet. "[I]n our study [we] have people self-rate their style of fighting to try to get to that issue," Bernick said. "Is the Floyd Mayweather–type fighter going to be okay, despite having forty-five or fifty fights? And a person who just goes straight ahead, a brawler, are they going to do worse if they've had the same number of fights and the same amount of training? You'd think that, but we don't have information on that yet so I don't know."

Until he dies and an autopsy is completed, there is nothing linking boxing to Benitez's prematurely painful demise or, for that matter, anyone else's. It's therefore helpful for boxers to donate their brains so research can be carried out on them. But many fighters have reservations about leaving their brains and a key part of their spinal cord behind. "A lot of the younger [fighters] aren't too excited by it, to be honest with you," Bernick says. "We do have some of the retired people who are interested and quite willing to do that because they're concerned. And sometimes having answers of why you're [behaving] a certain way can be consoling. . . . [I]t gives people closure and a sense of understanding [knowing] that's the cause."

MMA is a comparatively young sport, certainly in a mainstream capacity. And while fighters such as UFC veteran Gary Goodridge have discussed their problems and fears of CTE, the MMA fighters don't seem

(Spinks)

to be struggling in Bernick's study the same way the boxers are. Part of this is because MMA fighters often have had a superior education, so their starting point on some of the academic tests is higher. Part of it could also be because MMA fighters take fewer shots to the head given that they have so many other elements to work on, be it grappling, submissions, or strikes elsewhere to the body. Again, Bernick cannot confirm boxers are at greater risk; it's just that the study is leaning that way.

Bernick has made a breakthrough in Nevada, however. Because of the research at the Lou Ruvo Center, the Nevada State Athletic Commission now makes all of its athletes undergo a test to help track brain function over time. It marks the first time in sporting history that a regulatory body in any sport has followed brain function through the course of a career. It's only one state in a worldwide sport, but it's a start.

The answers to the questions researchers need remain buried in the brains of active and retired fighters, although Bernick is hopeful about breakthroughs. "[T]he most important findings are on the MRI side, that you can detect change over time and detect specific areas of the brain that seem vulnerable or are good markers of injury. . . . We can actually see the change based on how [the fighters are] performing on some of the cognitive tests. The thought is we eventually will find a way to track change and also, as we develop potential therapies, we'd like to be able to identify a group that's more likely to respond."

The Holy Grail is a biological marker of when a fighter should retire before it's too late. For now, though, Bernick believes that those surrounding a boxer should be well aware of the exposure he or she has had to punishment.

The Lou Ruvo Center's client list includes former heavyweight champion Leon Spinks, late former middleweight contender Joey Giambra, members of the Mayweather family, former light-heavyweight challenger John Scully, the brothers Jesse and Diego Magdaleno, ex-Olympian Tony Jeffries, and hundreds more.

Another is former WBO super-bantamweight champion Bones Adams. "Listen, I love Bernick," said the forty-five-year-old Adams, who trains fighters in Las Vegas. "He's a tremendous guy. He's a great guy to talk to and stuff. He's seen me, he knows the depression and stuff and I used to go there every month. . . . I wish I'd signed up for it earlier and I'd found out about it earlier so I could see, say, if I was fifteen years old, to see where I would be when I was twenty-five years old. The only thing I feel there's a change in is my speech, and I think the speech has to do with the energy. I have no energy, I'm fatigued all the time."

There are many challenging parts to Bernick's role in the program. He finds it hard when fighters come in and they are already symptomatic and it is even harder when they expect him to be able to both diagnose an illness and change or reverse their condition.

"We just don't have the tools yet," Bernick said, adding that more research needs to be completed and validated and that more clinical trials are required.

"This is where we are, this is the reason for the study," he explains. "We will help you out in any way, we're not just probing away, we will do whatever we can to help the fighter, but that's just the limitation. . . . At the moment we can't do anything to modify the disease itself. We can focus on treating symptoms and improving [the boxers'] function, but with the underlying disease, there's nothing we can do."

9

Contradiction

A NEUROLOGIST AT RINGSIDE

It's a few blocks from where the Cocoa Kid pleaded with people to spare him some change. Weill Cornell Medical Center in Manhattan is made up of several towering buildings that form a campus and takes up a vast amount of real estate along the East River.

On East 68th Street, six floors up in the Starr building is the neurology department, where Dr. Nitin Sethi works as the associate professor of clinical neurology. Sethi's list of qualifications is impressive. Born upstate in Buffalo, both his parents were doctors; his father specialized in neurology, his mother in pediatrics. He earned his medical degree from Maulana Azad Medical College at the University of Delhi and completed a residency in internal medicine in India. He moved back to New York in 2003, this time to the city, and was certified by the American Board of Psychiatry and Neurology (ABPN) and held integral positions for several neurophysiology organizations.

Cricket and soccer were the sports of Sethi's childhood, but in New York he tried a boxing class and was hooked. In fact, he enjoyed it so much that he decided to combine his passions of medicine and boxing, joining the New York State Athletic Commission in 2010 and becoming its chief medical officer in 2016. Having seen a lot of boxing in the gym, and having dealt with traumatic brain injuries and concussions for more than a decade, Sethi saw it as a natural fit. He earned a seat on the board of directors of the Association of Ringside Physicians and currently works as a medical officer at ringside. In a relatively short time, he began to wield some influence when it came to boxing, concussions, and long- and short-term brain injuries.

Meanwhile, Sethi has started work on a study titled "Quantifying Traumatically-Induced Neuroinflammation." According to the enrollment form, the purpose of the study is to see if new imaging tests can detect the effects of being hit on the head when standard tests do not. Specifically, it will look for inflammation in the brain after concussion.

"Most people who sustain a concussion recover without any long-term effects; however, some do not recover completely," he said.

While many medical organizations, including the British Medical Association, have called for boxing's abolition, Sethi is a neurologist who swims against the tide. "[The medical associations] say no amount of boxing is good for the brain," Sethi stated. "The way I feel the boxing community needs to go is, first and foremost, to identify and acknowledge the risk of boxing. And I'm talking about neurological injuries predominantly because . . . it's the acute traumatic brain injuries that are going to cause the unfortunate outcomes. If you really take the definitions of concussions, mild concussions—the word they use is subconcussive injuries— at face value, then they have subconcussive injuries during the rounds and they continue to box. As a neurologist, I'm acutely aware of that because that's what I do for a living. But maybe the boxing community doesn't understand. Education is still lacking. You don't need to have a dramatic KO for the fight to be stopped if he's been concussed. You might make the argument that if you start stopping the fight for every subconcussive injury in boxing then boxing will never exist in its current form. Think of it as probable TBI [traumatic brain injury], minor TBI, moderate to severe TBI. . . . The initial symptoms of a TBI in the ring . . . are all subjective. A headache is always subjective. I can't feel your headache. You have to say, 'I have a headache.' So headache, dizziness, nausea [are] all subjective. Obviously if you throw up I can see that. Then there are problems with focusing, double vision. . . . So if you have a doctor ringside, even if you're a neurologist, you can't really identify the initial onset unless a fighter says, 'Hey, I'm not feeling well.' When you get hit or you bump your head and you walk into a hospital, you say, 'Hey, I bumped my head, I don't feel well, I feel dizzy.' In boxing the culture has become, 'I'm not hurt. Shake it off. Fight on.' Which is fine. But then the community, which includes the doctors, needs to acknowledge that there are risks to that. . . ."

A key question often asked in boxing is this: when is the right time to stop a fight? It's widely understood that the referee is in the best position but a split second can change everything and no two people have the same view of a fight.

So what is the difference between a correct medical stoppage and a wrong one?

"A good medical stoppage is done at the right time, for the right medical indication," Sethi said. "If you stop a fight too early, if you stop a fight too late, if you stop a fight for the wrong medical indication, like a cut which is obviously not causing any problems, it's a bad medical stoppage and you are depriving a boxer, his team, of the fruits of their labor and the hours they've spent in the gym. You should be penalized; you should be criticized for that. . . . [W]hen it comes to TBI and concussion, I think one thing that should be acknowledged across the board—including by the fans who love this sport—you'd rather have the fight stopped a second too early rather than a second too late. That is the only way you can make boxing safe, because to make a medical call, which is [essentially] based on subjective complaints unless the patient talks to you, in this case the boxer, and they acknowledge, 'Yes, I'm hurt,' you have nothing to go on."

Sethi has made one infamous call. In 2019, as the ringside doctor at UFC 244, he pulled Nate Diaz out of a huge fight with Jorge Masvidal. Fans had anticipated a war at Madison Square Garden, but Sethi stopped the fight as it was heating up. He was doing his best to keep Diaz, who was cut and had been shaken, safe. He called it "a tough medical decision" but in the days that followed he was attacked online. After eighteen years of work and with a sound reputation, he received fake reviews on his medical internet profiles and people called his office, threatening him and his colleagues.

Sethi supervises club shows in Brooklyn or big bills at the Garden. His neurological colleagues think he's a contradiction and can't understand why he's interested in the sport, but Sethi can have the final word about who appears on a card and when a contest is ended. What happens on fight night can alter what happens to a boxer in the future. A bad beating or knockout can change the trajectory of a fighter's life.

What's more, boxers are taught to lie. They learn to feign being fine when they're tired or hurt. They can't admit to their opponent that they're feeling the pace of the contest or show that a punch has registered. Whether bloody, beaten, or not, they must remain stoic. When the referee asks if they're okay to continue, they must nod or face accusations of cowardice. That's the culture. It's a macho sport and a hard life.

But it's that philosophy that medical experts want to challenge. Sethi, who self-published the 2019 book *Neurologist at Ringside*, wrote a medical paper a year earlier titled "Can Boxing Be Made Safer? Yes, But the Culture Needs to Change." In it, he cited the instance of Roberto Duran turning his back on Sugar Ray Leonard in their 1980 rematch, which has since been labelled as the "No Más" fight. Duran was losing and, although perhaps not badly damaged, got frustrated and bailed out. The Panamanian, as great as he was, never fully lived it down but that is why the sport must change. "'When in doubt, sit it out' is not equivalent to 'no más,'" Sethi wrote. "'For he that fights and walks away may live to fight another day,' historically attributed to Demosthenes, a Greek orator, should be the new mantra of boxing. There is no shame in this; just [intelligence]."

He thinks a lot of it boils down to education and believes the NFL has been getting it right while boxing's macho façade remains stubbornly resolute. There does not have to be a loss of consciousness for a concussion to occur. NFL players would be benched after a heavy hit while it would be frowned upon for wanting respite in a prizefight

Sethi said: "[T]he culture has changed in football where if you feel you're concussed, . . . they have a neurologist or neurosurgeon at every game, one on the home side, one on the visitor's side, and the doctors are trained to identify these subtle concussions and to bring the player out. The player goes into the locker room, they give him a battery of tests including a neurological examination . . . if he's concussed he's benched. Boxing is unique. You don't have the luxury of doing a fifteen-minute examination on the sidelines. You either say the fight gets stopped or you let the fight continue."

Indeed, boxers have scraped themselves off the canvas, risen on wobbly legs, convinced a referee they have been okay to continue, and not only fought on but won. No in-fight examination. No halftime. Then back to war, with fans either screaming for their demise or for a miraculous rally. Sometimes fighters are so buzzed they don't remember what happened in the fight. They manage to compete on autopilot until they emerge through a fog. The medical term for that is post-traumatic amnesia. A fighter becomes amnestic after taking a headshot and for several minutes, or perhaps even longer, they can't recall what's happened. But because of a boxer's ability to fight on through that traumatic phase, Sethi admits that stopping fights for every subconcussive injury is "not practical."

In New York, referees and doctors are allowed to stop a contest, but in many states and countries only the referee is allowed. Sethi reckoned that empowering medical staff encouraged them to learn more about the sport and the boxers they are looking after.

He also believes trainers should educate fighters more about safety as they are on the front line and it has to come from the grass roots upward. The boxing media also has to play a role, he says, by not just highlighting tragedies but showing how to make them more preventable.

Something that will invariably help improve safety is national and global commissions sharing information. That a fighter may be suspended in one state on medical grounds but allowed to box elsewhere is crazy to everyone outside of boxing, yet it's commonplace. For example, Argentina's Hugo Alfredo Santillan was twenty-three when he took a bad beating in Germany on June 15, 2019, losing widely on points. He fought a draw on July 20 in San Nicolas, Argentina, when he was still serving a forty-five-day ban in Germany due to expire on July 30. He died from his injuries in the July 20 contest on July 25.

Yet unifying boxing at any level for the greater good has proved to be an impossible task.

Sethi wants a database that authorized officials can access that would include medical records, archived brain scans, and MRIs that paint an overall picture of a boxer's health.

"How you create that database is where the challenge is," Sethi admitted. "Who creates it? Who maintains it? But I think that sort of medical database should be there and people who love boxing—promoters, big promoters who have power and a say in boxing, governing bodies, big commissions—I think they have to join hands and say the medical aspect has to be [separated] from everything else. This is not turf war. . . . And the doctors should be independent. Doctors can't be aligned with different bodies."

But Sethi knows this is far off. In his 2017 paper, "Neuroimaging in Contact Sports: Determining Brain Fitness Before and After a Bout" he listed seventeen American commissions that all had different licensing requirements. In states like Arkansas, Florida, Illinois, and Arizona, you do not even need a radiological or neurological exam to box. In Nevada you only need an MRI or MRA (magnetic resonance angiography) scan, but it can be done without contrast, while California requires an MRI that needs previous scans to be compared with. In New Jersey, a fighter needs to have a radiological exam—a CT or MRI of the brain—which is valid for three years, while in Maryland a boxer needs a neurological exam, which has to be completed before his or her first bout and doesn't need to be renewed.

It is a cacophony of different standards and regulations and allows fighters to put their health on the line while almost everyone, perhaps even the boxer, remains oblivious to the risks.

Sethi wonders whether scans should be carried out on fighters immediately after each bout but then there's the radiation exposure to consider if someone is boxing multiple times each year.

Again, boxing's haphazard structure does not support any kind of regular tests. Unlike the NFL, there is no season in boxing, and therefore there is no off-season. Some boxers starting out may fight five or six times a year while those at the top may fight once or twice. Some may have had long training camps and sparred hundreds of rounds only to be injured and then unable to fight. Just because they don't make it to the contest, it doesn't mean there was no wear and tear on the brain from sparring. Everyone is different in terms of how much they spar, how often they fight, and how much damage they either take or are prone to.

And then, of course, should a fighter make it to that lofty level where one or two fights a year more than pays the bills, by that point their back catalog of bouts may include thirty or forty fights and anywhere between twenty and hundreds of amateur contests and thousands of sparring rounds. Although they are fighting less, they have taken more.

Serial imaging seems to be the most helpful way forward, and not only would that aid fighters during their career it would help them decide when enough is enough, giving them images they can't argue with and preventing ill-fated comebacks.

"If the MRI starts showing changes, something significant, these are healthy, young people, their brain MRI should not be showing evidence of white matter disease, so that's important," Sethi stated. "When I stop doing this I want to look back and say, 'I did the right thing at the time with the knowledge I had.' Because new knowledge is coming out. The risk of CTE is now more apparent. CTE is not a new disease. It's not something unique to football."

There is also a neurocognitive evaluation that fighters can complete, a computer-based test that takes just fifteen minutes but can look at attention, concentration, memory, short-term memory, and verbal memory. Fighters taking the test would thus have a baseline at the start and it could be tracked when the test is repeated, raising a red flag if there's a decline.

One way of improving the sport could be to increase post-fight evaluations after a contest, whether it's with a brief cognitive iPad test or with mandated brain scans.

Sethi contends that CT scans would be easier to do simply because they are available everywhere. Not all hospitals have MRI scanners and a CT image can detect blood, which is what a doctor would be looking for immediately after a bout. Also, a CT scan can be completed in five minutes whereas an MRI takes twenty.

MRIs still have their place, clearly, because it's a more comprehensive scan and it can show prior hemorrhages and scarring.

To do them, fighters would have to postpone victory celebrations and losers would need to be enticed out of their defeated cocoons. Would they want to do it? Would they lie and say they felt fine to go on their way, or would they feel okay but maybe not yet be able to feel any kind of damage because of the adrenaline of the fight?

Again, it goes back to Sethi's key point: that fighters, their teams, and their families must be honest. But at what point does that integrity need to show itself? In a fight, if they get shaken or hurt, should they raise their hand and quit, saying they fear they have a concussion?

"I don't know that [a fighter quitting] is the best-case scenario given the history of boxing, given the nature of the sport, but I don't think it's inappropriate," Sethi reasoned. "I don't think the fighter should be ridiculed for it [stopping fighting] or feel he did not do the right thing. I think the emphasis is to educate and say, 'Listen, if you feel you're not okay, err on the side of caution. Let the doctors and neurologist check you out and if you feel you're not well, there's no shame in saying, 'I can't go forward. I will come back the next day.'"

Sethi admitted he didn't have the answers but reverts to the change required in the culture. Once a brain injury starts, there is nothing a ringside doctor can do. The best-case scenario is to get a fighter to a hospital alive and in front of a neurosurgeon.

And even from a trained eye, Sethi said it's hard to detect a brain injury because they take time to develop and appear. Maybe it takes an hour, maybe it's longer or perhaps it's more sudden.

Sethi explained: "I was at the Academy of American Neurology a few years ago and an Army doctor presented a paper and said, 'I see patients coming to the end of their time. These are veterans, and they say, 'After the war I've had attention problems, concentration problems, memory problems, agitation, aggressiveness, I can't hold down a job.' And they are labelling them as PTSD [post-traumatic stress disorder].' But if you look at these symptoms, those are the same symptoms you have when you have repeated concussions or post-concussion syndrome. In medicine things are not black-and-white; they are always gray."

That is perhaps where Sethi's outlook on boxing sits. He's aware that he presents a contradiction to his medical peers as a neurologist who works in boxing, and who also handles MMA assignments. In fact, he is more at ease watching MMA because of victories coming through submissions, tap-outs, and not every fighter looking for head strikes to win a fight.

He is also open to other practical suggestions that might help boxing, such as revisiting glove size, the number of rounds and their duration, and headgear. But, for now, it is during fight night when he can make a difference. Even if he is not saving lives in the strictest sense, he can help preserve the quality of them down the line. And there are changes he believes he can instigate that will benefit fighters.

As things stand, any kind of physician can work at ringside. You might have a neurologist but you could also have an orthopedic specialist.

"Do you mandate that among the three or four ringside doctors assigned to a fight that one of them has studied the neurosciences?" Sethi pondered. "Either a neurologist or a neurosurgeon? That's a practical suggestion. I've thought about things that are more outside the box. I sometimes hear the commentators talking about the fight and they're so knowledgeable; they are watching the punches better than us because they're looking at the screen right in front of them. I've also thought about that, if they somehow gave us a signal and said, 'Listen, we have seen something on the screen you guys might not have noticed. I think you should stop the fight.' There's no harm in having that communication come through. I'm not sure how that would work and I'm not saying they should influence fights, but, again, in football, a hit happened, you see the hit on the big screen, and on the sideline you miss the hit. That's why they have spotters who are trained who can call down and say, 'I saw the hit.' And they can go back and forth and see it clearly. I'm not trained like commentators are and they see these things better than me. It's a second pair of eyes seeing the fight and I'm hearing what their thoughts are."

Sethi made sure it was known he is speaking only on his behalf, not that of the Athletic Commission he works on. But the Athletic Commission should listen to his words as he strives to make the sport safer.

But how can a sport as chaotic as boxing create wholesale changes?

"We choose our professions and every profession has its hazards," Sethi concluded. "They are professional athletes. Acknowledging the risks of boxing doesn't mean you're giving it a negative image."

Sethi's ideas— a centralized database, doctors who know the sport and boxers thoroughly, improved scans, and the change in culture—seem a long way off. Not all neurologists want the sport abolished, as contradictory as that might be to their own backgrounds and their own community. Boxing needs to embrace those who want to help it. Sethi might not have all of the answers, but he wants what is best for boxing, and anyone with a brain will tell you that's a good thing.

10
Chaos

BOXING'S ENDLESS PROBLEM

"The problem is that it's always been an issue, it remains an issue, and it will continue to be an issue as we go forward because people are getting hit in the head."

Dr. Margaret Goodman, who has seen plenty of damaged and deteriorating fighters, has been involved in boxing for more than twenty years. She was on the medical board of the Nevada State Athletic Commission and then, disenfranchised with boxing and its internal workings, made a break and launched the Voluntary Anti-Doping Association (VADA), which is widely viewed as the premier drug-testing agency in boxing and combat sports. During her time on the commission, fighters came and went. She became close to some. She also saw them change and she saw how boxing changed them.

She has also been changed by her experiences and has become hardened. She still cares—about the sport and about fighters—but there is more resignation than enthusiasm in her voice. It comes to a lot of fight people after years of disappointment. She has seen "shot" fighters, punch-drunk fighters, and she has watched them degenerate. She has even seen some receive licenses to fight, knowing their health and futures were at risk. She has witnessed young, ambitious pros become old mumbling relics.

"It hurts me terribly," she said. "I mean, we can go back years and years ago when we were stopping certain fighters from competing and it just hurts your heart. We would show them the deterioration in person and say, 'This is how you were. This is how you are now. Do you see the change?' And they wouldn't see it. But they didn't want to and it breaks you but you can't make them understand."

She has seen a fading boxer's life come off the rails, a story so familiar it's on a loop. It is not just the depression that comes when a career winds down. Life in the limelight becomes life in the dull gloom of retirement. Many are damaged, and that is accentuated by the loss of their career. And while there are physical signs in fighters, there is plenty more we do not see behind closed doors that wives, partners, and children of broken fighters live with. "These athletes aren't getting adequately treated and what happens at home with these fighters after a fight or between fights?" asked Goodman. "People might say, 'Oh, he lost a fight, he's depressed' or 'He doesn't have a fight coming up, he's depressed.' It's a vicious cycle. I think [American] football probably has all of these analogies and situations, which have been written about much more."

Goodman was referring to the likes of Mike Webster, Junior Seau, and Dave Duerson. Seau was just forty-three when he committed suicide. Later studies concluded that he too suffered from CTE. Before he passed, Duerson, a father of four, left a suicide note pleading for his brain to be left to the brain bank so researchers could find out what had been happening to him. The answers were never available when he was alive, so he hoped people might be able to understand in death. "Please, see that my brain is given to the NFL's brain bank," he wrote. He had shot himself in the chest to preserve his brain. Seau also shot himself in the chest.

Of course, there have been many similar cases in boxing over the last hundred years. They were mostly greeted by a shrug of the shoulders and a single word with a simplistic and insulting connotation: "punchy."

In 2001, Goodman—through the Nevada State Athletic Commission—released a book titled *Ringside and Training Principles*. It was a one-stop shop for fighters, providing them with information about diet, workouts, making weight, the business side of boxing, advice for amateurs, dealing with cuts, the use of drugs and alcohol, regulations, and even financial counsel. Goodman wrote a chapter called "Acute and Chronic Head Injuries: How to Lengthen Your Career and Perhaps Save Your Life" and opens it powerfully: "People, especially doctors frequently ask me, 'How can you, a neurologist, a brain doctor, work in boxing?' It seems like a morbid fascination to many physicians. In truth, I have learned about being a better neurologist from my work with fighters and trainers. No one can debate genetics, skill, and luck in preventing head injuries. To some degree, I believe they can be avoided through a better understanding of how they occur."

Then, she focuses directly on the fighter/reader: "When you are at the end of your career, there is no one there to protect you. It sounds harsh, but eventually everyone retires from the ring. Whether it is after one fight or fifty, what you have left has to be your responsibility. Whether you can hold a job, raise a family, own a company, or carry on a conversation is up to YOU!"

Goodman discusses acute head injuries, describing how the brain shifts in the skull upon the impact of a punch. She talks about brain bleeds, how blows can cause a tear or stretch of a vessel that connects the brain and its coverings, resulting in a clot or bleed. "The more rotation the skull undergoes, the greater the potential for injury and loss of consciousness," she writes.

She clarifies that a loss of consciousness does not have to happen for a concussion to occur and grades concussions on a scale of 1 to 3. A grade 1 concussion is when there is no amnesia and no loss of consciousness. A grade 2 concussion is when there is confusion, amnesia concerning the fight or the events surrounding it, but still no loss of consciousness. Grade 3 is a loss of consciousness. She writes that headaches are often a "hallmark of concussion" and adds "LET ME RESTATE THIS FOR EMPHASIS: Someone can function with a concussion but continuing to take punishment with one can lead to permanent brain damage."

She opens her section on chronic injuries with a warning. "The most difficult aspect of chronic brain injuries lies in the mere fact that by the time a fighter is showing symptoms, it's too late."

We still do not have answers to a lot of the questions surrounding how a fighter's brain becomes chronically compromised, but Goodman states that variables include the number of fights, the number of knockouts, the sparring regime, how good the boxer was and whether he or she declined, and the use of drugs and alcohol. First symptoms of brain injury, she notes, are slowed reflexes, slurred or garbled speech, memory loss and confusion, fatigue, difficulty with balance, and personality changes, be it paranoia or mood swings. Goodman has witnessed them all firsthand. Unfortunately for boxing's sake, her beliefs and values do not align with the sport's power brokers or their economic goals.

Goodman also argues it is important that the medical people in the sport are also boxing people because they would have seen fighters transition through their careers and seen their decline. They would not be assessing a fighter blind, meeting them for the first time in their office and giving the fighter a standard test to pass in order to get licensed.

"There was a fighter who was very successful who fought Marco Antonio Barrera, who fought a lot of people, lived in New York, and he had really tough fights," said Goodman. "I remember getting a call from a TV company and I said, 'Listen, I think this guy really is in trouble. I've seen him in the gym.' We knew he was going to fight out of Nevada, so we said, 'You need to have this thorough exam.' We sent him to one of the most prominent behavioral neurologists in New York and that guy passed him. He said, 'Well, he looks good to me.' Meanwhile, the guy was really in trouble. His gait was off, his coordination was off, I knew his cognitive functioning was off too as part of what people told me, and it was terrible. And we had to allow him to fight because we didn't have the documentation to make the determination. One of the reasons I left the commission was because I wasn't able to make that determination, to say even though the tests are normal this guy is in trouble and should not be licensed. It was just too frustrating. There would be a fighter fighting in New Jersey and he was going to box in Nevada and I could see from the films how this guy no longer looked good, but meanwhile he was allowed to go fight somewhere because no one could see the deterioration in his functioning in the ring."

It sounds all too familiar: A fighter is refused a license, so he gets one elsewhere. A fighter is suspended on a drug violation, so he fights elsewhere. A fighter is banned on a disciplinary measure, so he fights elsewhere. The lack of unity between the governing and sanctioning bodies makes boxing sport's Wild West. This is the way it has always been. Whether you're in the Nevada State Athletic Commission or the

British Boxing Board of Control or if you're part of the Luxembourg Boxing Federation or under the auspices of the New York State Athletic Commission, the playing fields are different. Will anything change?

"I can't, in my lifetime, imagine that's possible," Goodman lamented. "In the United States and worldwide, no one wants to give up their piece of the pie, irrespective of what the repercussions are to the fighters. That's one aspect I battled for many, many years. In the years before [Senator] John McCain got ill, he was trying to have a national [boxing] commission and everyone would have to follow the same rules. People said they wanted it, but they were pushing hard behind the scenes so it wouldn't happen, because they didn't want to give up their control. It's not necessarily because of tax income, which is really why a commission is created in the United States. It's for the tax that comes to the state so it's not to protect the fighters. They may say it's to protect the fighters but it just isn't. I don't care what they would say. Number one is money. Number two it's to protect the politicians who oversee the state, to protect the government. Number three may be to protect the fighters, and that's the way it is in every state. In most states, at least in the U.S., the bottom line is often the person running the commission office has no real knowledge of boxing or MMA. They wouldn't know if someone was hurt if you punched them in the head to show [them] what it was like."

But would organizations not get on the same page for the sake of the boxers, the ones in the firing line? Goodman counters that promoters want to have the ability to take their fighters elsewhere, regardless of why they might not have been licensed by a governing body.

"It's frustrating because these people really are meat to them," she said. "I understand it. It's a two-way street. If there weren't boxing promoters, there wouldn't be fights. If there weren't fighters, there wouldn't be boxing promoters. It's a symbiotic relationship, but the bottom line is how much do they really care about that fighter? How much do they care about the opponent they are putting in with that fighter? How many Mexican fighters have been brought over to build boxing cards as opponents? And how many commissions that bring fighters over from foreign countries know if that fighter has slurred speech or if they're really able to understand the fighter they're assessing because they don't understand the fighter's accent? There are those issues, it's just a multitude of problems that doesn't really get repaired. If you can't enforce things, people just aren't going to do it. It's really hard with the sport being so disjointed."

Then there's the political side of who is assigned to work a fight from an officiating aspect. Who works ringside? Who evaluates the fighters in the locker rooms? Do they have enough experience? And who's not afraid, because sometimes the right call is not the most popular call.

"The problem is—and everyone has their own ax to grind—but as a former ringside physician, if you stop a fight or recommend a fight should be stopped from a promoter that has big connections with the commission, you're never going to work another fight again," Goodman said. "Same thing for the referees. Same thing for the judges. It looks like everybody cares, but they only care so much because otherwise they wouldn't be there. The politics involved in the sport is probably just as important as the actual head trauma the fighters are taking because people don't want to step on other people's toes. There are too many outside influences, and so the overall health of the sport has not improved as much as it could from those factors as well, which most people don't take into account."

Goodman also argued that the officials who work fights are not necessarily trained well enough with respect to brain injury, and there's certainly no supervision in gyms. That is another fight in itself, she admitted, but certainly if ringside physicians, officials, and referees are not trained well enough to recognize when someone's having problems it compounds the issue.

So who should be charged with looking after the boxers on fight night? "In some respects a neurologist isn't the right person," Goodman continued. "In some respects an emergency room physician might be the best person to have on site. Another problem is when the ringside physicians don't do a good job in helping the referee make a determination, nobody says anything. They may mention it on television, but the commissions might not do anything about it. They might do something on a poor performance of a judge. People may criticize the referee. Nobody ever criticizes the physicians. Physicians that do a bad job should not be involved, and there're plenty of them and no one does anything to stop that. It's a very different education to acquire, and too many doctors think they know everything, and that's a problem too. It's annoying when people sitting there can determine that this shouldn't be going on, yet the ring officials are allowing it to continue for a number of reasons and there's a whole bunch of things that go into that. I get it. Trust me, I know. It's hard to stop something, but some of these things go on too long."

Of course, Goodman has worked with fighters at the highest level from Floyd Mayweather to Wladimir Klitschko and Oscar De La Hoya to James Toney but habits are often formed when young boxers are amateurs and picking up new things. Certainly they're sparring young and taking plenty of trauma before they even turn pro and Goodman would like to see a more thorough record kept of an amateur boxer's career. She's had to assess fighters while being unable to tell how many bouts they'd had and what the outcomes of those contests were.

"All those rounds count," she said. "Sparring rounds as well, oh my God."

It's not just the start of a fighter's career when they need to be looked after but at the end, too. Take Wilfred Benitez, for example, who near the end of his career lost to the likes of Carlos Herrera, Pat Lawlor, and Scott Papasodora. He was clearly no longer the fighter he had been in his prime. His peak was early but was realistically his career was over by his mid-twenties.

Yet some fighters improve in their thirties while a few have thrived in their forties. There is no pattern and no one knows how much punishment is too much.

"To put some kind of arbitrary number on it [the amount of fights a boxer has] would be silly, but I think that fighters don't need to spar nearly as much," Goodman added. "Look at Floyd Mayweather. Floyd was a gym rat, continues to be a gym rat, but doesn't spar much. So that's a shining example of the way a fighter should be. But that is not always the case and I'm sure he sparred a ton when he was younger—but he sparred less and less as he went on, even though he was in the gym always training. The other bottom line is that fighters don't stay in shape and that's another thing that causes this up and down in their weight or their eating or taking care of themselves. This is a career and if they're going to do it they need to treat it as a career and not a hobby. Too many fighters do that."

There are more gray areas. How can you tell one fighter to retire at the age of thirty while another may be setting out on his journey at the same age? When should those in attendance on fight night stop a one-sided fight? When has a boxer absorbed too much punishment? Is it up to the fighter to say? Is it up to the trainer, the referee, or the doctor? And why shouldn't a boxer be allowed to fight to the brink when heroes like

Philadelphia legend Matthew Saad Muhammad and New Jersey slugger Arturo Gatti could take round after round of abuse before battling back, repeatedly capturing unlikely victories?

"There are so many fighters who are hurt in a fight and come back to win, and that's another problem," Goodman continued. "So many commissions look at the fighter who just lost, they may not look at the fighter who won, not thinking he might be in just as much trouble as the one who lost. He might be in much more trouble than that one, but how many regulatory bodies really look at that person? They may not have to because he's got a W by his name."

Then, of course, it is not in the short term that the effects of a boxing career are seen but in the long term. Gatti died in 2009 in suspicious circumstances at the age of thirty-seven. Many believed he would have struggled with poor health after so many wars, but we never got to find out. We did with Saad Muhammad. His speech was slurred, he walked as though he was wearing magnetic boots, and his short-term memory was impaired. Saad lost his money, then he lost his friends, and then he lost his health. Whether those who made the final examinations of his body knew he was a boxer and that they should have been looking for CTE is unknown but it should have been checked for.

The long-term damage associated with boxing is something Goodman has never shied away from and she says it's "a real problem" but admits she doesn't know how to fix it—with the exception of stopping punches to the head.

And post-career, fighters will continue to struggle, some embarrassed by their conditions, some with families embarrassed that their once-fine fathers or grandfathers have been reduced to trembling, shuffling relics. "Nobody should be embarrassed by all these things but they kind of get pushed under the rug, and too many families of people who are working with these fighters, for one reason or another, they don't say anything," Goodman offered.

It has been nearly two decades since the Nevada State Athletic Commission released *Ringside and Training Principles*. Since then, the NFL continued to explore different options and safety measures. It might have taken a while but changes have been made. And more is also being done in other sports to help their stars and players. Yet boxing still occupies a time in the dark ages.

"The whole purpose of the book was to educate the fighters," Goodman stated. "The commissions . . . you can't really change. You can make them change if somebody dies or if they get a lot of media attention they'll do it. If it's in the *New York Times* they'll do it, to some degree. But the fighters themselves have to make the change. And I tend to believe—and this is kind of idealistic—that most of these fighters are very smart. No one gives them credit. They say, 'Oh, they didn't have the education. . . . They didn't finish college. . . . That they're not smart.' But they're smart. You have to be smart to be a boxer, to be a successful boxer."

It is not just the fighters who come out of the sport damaged. While Goodman remains a force for good as the head of VADA, it's clear the sport has taken a toll on her. Fighter safety will always be paramount, but it is sad to think that is one of the reasons why she is on the outside looking in. It's sad that, until only recently, she has not even been able to watch a fight on TV because she gets "too annoyed."

Boxing had left her with a severe case of burnout. It can happen when someone cares too much and spends their time shouting when no one cares to listen.

"I hadn't watched a fight for a while even though I do still love the sport," she concluded. "I was at the gym and there was an afternoon fight on television and the referee and the doctor had done just a crappy job and the fighter suffered a severe injury, I don't think he died but I think he was terribly disabled, had to have brain surgery and I was thinking, 'Why am I watching this?' I hadn't watched a fight in about five years. This was the one fight I watched. Did that fight change anything? No. Did that commission do anything different? No. Did they like the headlines that they got for about five days afterward? No. But where was the money or the initiative to really make a change? When I was on the commission I used to say, 'We need to make changes now. We need to stop accepting falsified medical tests. . . .' This [Nevada] commission did make changes. Has it made things safer? They'd argue yes. In the short term maybe it did. Did it affect the long term?"

Has anything affected the long term? Will it ever? Is punch-drunk syndrome a curse, something that will command little more than a shrug of the shoulders, a shake of the head, a GoFundMe page, or a sigh? Goodman's skepticism is well-placed. Things haven't changed for fighters over the years. Why would they now? Even with Dr. Charles Bernick's study in Las

Vegas and the research being undertaken in Boston, will boxing allow any discoveries to be made relevant, to be of any use to the fighters? Is there an interest within the sport to change?

Goodman sees what Dr. Bernick and the others are trying to do, but wonders whether it would affect the greater good of the sport. "That's one of the things the Lou Ruvo Center is trying to do," she said. "But how much of that documentation is being shared with the commission? I remember asking Dr. Bernick a long time ago when they started their study [that] if someone's got a serious problem, like they've got a bleed on their brain or they've got an aneurysm, can you tell the commission that? They said no. Obviously they could ask the fighter if they wanted them to tell the commission, but if the fighter says no they can't say anything because the fighter is involved with the study. And even if they were the fighter's physician, they would have the law [client-patient confidentiality] where they couldn't release that information. It's a real problem because there's no sharing of information. Long-term [damage] is a bigger issue than many think."

She knows boxers who have had elocution lessons to improve their worsening speech in retirement. England's Jimmy Batten, famous for a 1982 decision defeat to Roberto Duran in Miami, had them and even wound up with some acting parts.

"Lou Ruvo have added taping the fighters' speech pattern, because that's obviously something that deteriorates pretty quickly—that could be adequate for them to make a determination, but I don't know how the information is being shared," Goodman added. "Maybe it's being shared better. It's just an endless problem."

Goodman, for so long a friend to fighters, looked coldly at the sport's landscape. She knows it all too well. "The question is, what is all this data and research accomplishing so far? I don't really know. I think it's all wonderful. It's kind of telling us what we always knew. Nobody studied it because there was no money in a study, but now we know all this stuff from this research. It's what we always knew from before, and trust me, I'm not someone who thinks boxing should be abolished, but knowing what we know now, should it be?" She laughed nervously.

What we do know is that unless things change, fighters won't be any healthier when they leave the ring for the final time.

11
Dilemma

A DAMAGED FIGHTER WONDERS WHETHER HE SHOULD TRAIN BOXERS

"I think the first thing you see go on a fighter is [their] legs, and when you see them go a little bit they have difficulty with timing. That's the biggest thing."

Trainer Freddie Roach was a contender when he fought through the early 1980s. Then one day he tripped while running and turned his ankle. He kept dragging the affected foot after that, it changed the way he moved around the ring, and other symptoms followed.

"My legs went two years before I was diagnosed with Parkinson's . . . and doing roadwork was almost impossible because sometimes my knee would bend and sometimes it wouldn't," Roach admitted.

He became a trainer, one of the best in the sport's history, working with more than twenty world champions, including Virgil Hill, Marlon Starling, Mike Tyson, Manny Pacquiao, James Toney, and Michael Moorer. He opened up his own Los Angeles gym, the Wild Card Boxing Club, which became one of the go-to venues in world boxing. He understands what goes on inside and outside the ropes, he gets the business, and he also knows the risks.

For a long time, Roach didn't believe his Parkinson's was related to his fighting career, or at least he didn't admit to that publicly. Now he sees things differently and accepts that boxing damaged him. He visits a neurologist regularly and his most visible symptoms have been an unsteady gait and at-times-violent hand tremors. He also has concerns about his short-term memory and, at sixty years old, he has seen some of his contemporaries struggle with neurological issues in retirement.

On the front line, he's also had to warn boxers about the dangers of fighting on too long or staying in the sport when it can do more harm than good. How do you tell a fighter that it's over or that they're "shot"?

"You'd probably be a little kinder in conversation about it," Roach began, prickling at the mention of being "shot," a label old fighters dread. "But when you're going to tell someone to retire and they ask why, you have to be able to give them reasons. Sometimes I see it in fighters that are not mine and I say, 'He's going to have problems later,' and it usually works out that way. But if it's not my fighter, it's surely not my business. I would love to try to help them but the thing is, once they 'go,' it's over. I know a fighter who's in my gym, he's a current world champion and he's been a pro for a long, long time and he's been in the gym a long, long time and his legs are starting to go a little bit. I've seen it in sparring and so forth. But since I don't train him, I really can't say much so I try not to use him as a sparring partner for my guys because I don't want my guys to hurt anybody. It's a very delicate procedure. I've told seven guys to retire in my lifetime . . . five told me to go and fuck myself."

The legendary Eddie Futch, one of the all-time great corner wizards, trained Roach, and being told you have to retire when it is all you know is not an easy thing to hear. Roach understands because Futch warned him. Roach told Futch to go fuck himself. Roach fought on, got beaten up, and lost four of his next five fights without Futch and then retired.

"Eddie told me, 'I think it's time to retire,'" Freddie recalled, having been told he was being hit too much. "I said, 'It's easy for you to say but it's all I know. What am I going to do?' He said, 'You'll find a job. You're a capable person.' And I said, 'You're pretty old yourself. Why don't you think about retiring?' I walked out. I was really upset when he told me. After that, I lost four of the five fights and then I went to Mr. Futch and I said, 'I'm sorry, I was wrong, you were right. I'm sorry I took those fights, I should have listened to you. I want to be your assistant and I want to help you.' He didn't say yes, but I started showing up every day. And every day I would do the bags and mitts with the fighters. Virgil Hill was the first one to ask me to do mitts with him and then Virgil became the first one to become champion. He left Eddie and stayed with me, he and Marlon Starling. For some reason they didn't get along as well with Mr. Futch as other people did, and they became my fighters and were my first two world champions."

While Roach's training stock rocketed, his health deteriorated. He has suffered with bad tremors and has also noted times when they have improved although he's been self-conscious of them when he has been on television. Muhammad Ali also experienced tremors, symptoms that are consistent with their Parkinson's diagnosis, but both also took a lot of punches.

Roach's late mother, Barbara, did not think Freddie's damage was boxing related.

"She thought I had Parkinson's because when I was a tree surgeon back when I used to work for my dad, we used to spray trees and yards with chemicals and we didn't know about it back then, there were no regulations. She thinks maybe it was some of the chemicals I was spraying being an arborist."

It was Roach's father who led him and his siblings into boxing. Roach's brother Pepper was particularly athletic and went on to become a pro boxer. "I wasn't as good an athlete as my brother Pepper was," Roach said, "but now he's had two strokes and he's not doing so well. He still works in my gym and he still remembers the past, but if you ask him what happened yesterday he'd have a tough time telling you." Pepper had ten professional fights but boxed far more rounds, in the amateurs and in sparring, spending his life in the sport.

"When I started boxing it was to make my father happy," Roach remembered, "to make him an easier dad to be around. [There were] five boys in my family and the eldest brother quit boxing at the age of fifteen because he didn't like it—so he got thrown out of the house. He had to quit school and get a job and actually he did very well for himself later in life in the petroleum business. But getting thrown out of the house at fifteen? Shit. He was staying at friends' houses who were still at high school and he then got a job that paid him enough money to pay the rent on a small apartment. . . . He doesn't have any neurological issues or anything like the three of us that boxed the most, Joey, Pepper, and me. . . . My youngest brother [Paul] didn't box because my mother had had enough of it with us by then."

It's a dilemma that has caused Roach to question what he does as a coach—working in a sport where he sees punches to the head on a daily basis. The Wild Card is infamous for its hard sparring.

"Maybe I'm wrong for teaching people the sport that maybe gave me the disease I have," Roach said. "Some people accuse me of being a hypocrite and I say, 'Well, it's what I know. I know the signs of it. I know the bad problems of it and I can see it better than you can, and I can see it faster than you can because I've lived it. I've been there.' Not all trainers will address [the problem of head trauma] though. Some trainers, some people in the world want to make a living and all they care about is the fucking payday. I'm different from that. I don't care about the payday, I care about the health of the fighter and I will do everything I can to see him safe."

There is not much Roach has not seen in nearly five decades in boxing and his own neurological issues make him sympathetic to his fighters. He says he listens to them and their concerns, adapting his training schedules as he's become more educated about the cumulative effect of head trauma. "My whole career I sparred six days a week. I sparred every day. Every day I trained, I sparred. Now I get guys who spar one day, I see the mistakes they made and what they need to improve on, I study the sparring and the next day on the mitts we practice what they need to improve on. I think six days a week was crazy, three days a week maybe—still pushing it a little bit—two days is better. Can you get away with not sparring? No, I don't think so. I think timing and distance and things of that nature have to be adjusted and can only be adjusted in sparring. We do need some sparring, yes, but we don't need ten rounds every day. I think fighters overspar and I think that has a lot to do with the problems."

Roach has taken the information from his own neurologists and has applied it as best he can. The research employed by the NFL has shaped his own views, too. He is all too aware of boxing's concussion crisis. "If you have a fighter who is getting ready for a big fight and he gets knocked out, he needs to have an MRI and go through all the tests [and] then you've got to be honest with him," Roach insisted. "But most trainers will just ignore it and give him a couple of days off sparring and back they go. . . . And it will show up when they're in the ring fighting. I think that's a trainer's responsibility, to make sure the fighter is going in there healthy."

Then there is the equipment, to protect the hands, the teeth, and, yes, the head. Again, with his more recent education, Roach's stance has softened toward the equipment his fighters use. "You know the headgear with the bar on the front?" he asked. "The first time Manny Pacquiao brought one of those I threw it in the garbage because I didn't think it would help with defense. The bar would protect the fighter too much. Then I started thinking about it and I do like it now because I think it prevents some injuries. . . . Getting ready for a world-title fight is very difficult. Most guys get injured. No one goes into a fight 100 percent in boxing. They all have some type of injury, the hand, a cut, or something. Equipment like that bar prevents them getting cut as much as anything. The defense can still be there and it can still be taught."

Doctors have told Roach that they suspect his illness has come from his fighting career, but he's been told it can't be proved. He's been assessed by some of the finest neurologists in the United States but it's not just his own fighters he has seen descend into poor health but rivals and contemporaries, too.

Bobby Chacon was one of them. Nicknamed "The Schoolboy" because of his young features, Chacon was a dashing featherweight who peaked in the late 1970s and early '80s. He was a classic TV fighter, involved in any number of famous boxing slugfests and the type of wars that shorten careers. All those memorable nights, against the likes of Rafael "Bazooka" Limon, Cornelius Boza-Edwards, and Ruben Olivares, had come at a heavy price, but he was adored for them.

Back before he retired, Chacon, like so many others, had fought on too long. Although he was still winning, he was doing so at a cost. His wife, Valerie, could see her husband changing. It was as if she knew what the future would hold. He was involved in war after war, becoming a promoter's dream and a fight fan's hero. She wanted him to bank his savings and grow old and happy with her and their three children. But Chacon, who had been the WBC featherweight champion, refused to walk away. Chacon still had blood to spill, memories to make, and a championship to win back. He wasn't done. Even as far back as 1976, after Chacon had been left battered and bruised by David Sotelo, Valerie had asked her husband to retire. For years she kept begging him and he kept not listening. On March 15, 1982, Valerie, only thirty-one years old, shot herself in the head.

Chacon fought again the very next night, against Salvador Ugalde, of Los Angeles. He won in three rounds. Even the fight's promoter, Bob Griffin, didn't think it was right to hold the card. He initially postponed the fight, only to reinstate it at Chacon's behest.

One of Chacon's late career victories came against a young pro out of Dedham, Massachusetts, Freddie Roach. Roach lost a majority decision over ten rounds, despite twice flooring Chacon in round two. Chacon finally retired in 1988. He'd been at it for sixteen years. A matinee idol, he was dead at the age of sixty-five having long suffered from dementia. He had won fifty-nine of sixty-seven fights, losing just seven and drawing one. In retirement he frequented the Wild Card Boxing Club and was the life and soul of the party wherever he went.

Roach saw Chacon often over the years that followed, Roach battling Parkinson's but still a successful trainer, Chacon toiling with dementia. It was sad for Roach to witness. He thought it had as much to do with Chacon's hard life away from the ring that resulted in his sad condition.

"Some of the fighters that are really shot, they have a disease first of all and they don't take care of their bodies second of all. A lot of guys are on drugs or alcohol—and when you mix these together [with] the sport of boxing you're really going to have a bigger problem and a more noticeable problem," Roach said. "Obviously Bobby was very noticeable. He seemed to be happy, yes, but he really didn't kind of know where he was and he was kissing everyone. I said, 'Remember when we fought?' and he said, 'Yeah, I knocked you out.' And I said, 'No, I knocked you down twice.' And he said that never happened. So he remembered the fight but he [was] a little bit delusional about his boxing career."

Roach, in becoming boxing's highest-profile trainer, had his own reality show on HBO. Many believe that in the TV show *Ray Donovan*, the character Terry—a retired fighter-cum-boxing coach in Hollywood with tremors—is based on him. Roach has had endorsements with Nike and Under Armour while celebrities such as Mark Wahlberg, Mickey Rourke, Mario Lopez, and Bob Dylan have all visited him at his Wild Card Boxing Club.

Roach remembers, with a particular fondness, the day one celebrity came in—Muhammad Ali. The two talked about things they had in common and the time flew by. "My tremors were noticeable then, they weren't violent but it's funny because when Muhammad Ali walked in my gym, he asked me if he could work out," Roach started. "And I was by myself, it was early in the morning and I said, 'Yes, sure.' Ali went in the dressing room, came out, and he went after the biggest bag in the gym—like a heavyweight is supposed to do—and I was happy about that. And as he started punching the bag his tremors went away. I said, 'Me and you have something in common.' He said, 'What's that?' I said, 'When you start hitting the heavy bag and hitting the combinations and so forth you don't shake anymore.' He said, 'Yeah, that's why I like hitting the bag.' I said, 'When I get in the ring and start catching punches [on the mitts], I don't shake either.'"

"It was interesting. I called my doctor and asked if there was any correlation to that and he said, 'It could be your comfort zone. It's what you're used to and it's what you're comfortable at and comfortable doing' and he said, 'It does open the book up a little bit if we can study it, to see if there's an answer to it.' But there's been no answer yet. Everyone is so different. When Ali came in that day, it was a little embarrassing with his tremors and I felt bad for him. He couldn't sign his autograph well. But he did some magic tricks and he was here for four hours and it was probably the best day I had in the gym. It changed my mind what kind of person he was because I was a Joe Frazier fan, my trainer [Eddie Futch] trained Frazier, of course, but after speaking to Ali for a while and getting his sense of humor, I was an Ali fan. He was very funny."

Roach is concerned about his memory and he also worries for MMA fighters, like Georges St-Pierre, who he has trained for several big fights.

"Fighters lie," he sighed. "You can't see concussions. The thing is, I think the physicals and the tests we have now are a lot better than when I was a fighter. They have MRIs now and they have to pass a lot more tests and I think that's good for the sport and I think that hopefully, maybe, it will eliminate some of the injuries. But in this sport, you're going to have injuries because it is somewhat a violent sport."

Despite spending three decades with Parkinson's, Roach has no regrets over his career. He has been more successful post-fighting and he has both fame and fortune. The one thing he missed was winning a world-title belt.

"I'm okay with my career," he concluded. "I didn't achieve my goal. I never became a world champion, so I feel like I failed in my dream. But I'm content and I've found a job now that I'm better at and I train fighters as best as I can, and I'm okay with that and I watch out for them the best I can also.

"With Parkinson's, sometimes you wake up and think, 'Why the fuck did they pick me?' But, you know, that's part of life. Some of the medications do cause depression and so forth and some mornings I'll think about bad things. But then I'll go to the gym and go to work and everything bad goes away. I told my neurologist that sometimes I think about killing myself. He asked me why and I said, 'It's just fucking difficult sometimes dealing with this shit.'"

It is not just the quick, sudden death Roach will watch out for, but the start of the long, slow one that comes to pass for so many. That is a corner he does not want to be in.

12
Buried Alive

"BOXING IS AMERICAN FOOTBALL HEAD INJURIES ON STEROIDS"

Denny and Phil Moyer's father bathed, washed, and fed his boys. He brushed their teeth. He did everything a parent should do. He walked arm in arm with them. He helped them find the words they could not locate. He looked after them and made sure they wanted for nothing. The problem was that Denny and Phil were adults. Both retired fighters, Denny was seventy and Phil was sixty-two. Their father, Harry, was ninety-five, and he had helped take care of them like this for over a decade.

The once-fabulous Moyer siblings muddled around the hallways of a nursing home in Oregon, confused. They wore bicycle helmets in case they fell, clung to metal frames while shuffling down empty corridors. When they stopped to talk, their conversations went around in circles, Harry not really knowing what to say and his children scarcely remembering how to speak.

Denny had far more fights than Phil. As a professional, he won ninety-eight times, lost thirty-eight, and drew four. He fought 1,302 professional rounds in 141 fights between 1957 and 1975.

Phil followed his older brother into the sport, though he did not have Denny's passion. He preferred football, but boxing was in the family. Their father and uncles boxed.[3] Their Uncle Tom had trained them. Phil had just thirty-eight fights and competed in 312 rounds. He won twenty-eight contests, lost nine, and drew one. Yet here he was, in the Gracelen Terrace Nursing Home in the same situation as his brother: desolate, hollow, numb, and helpless.

Throughout their careers, Denny and Phil had been handsome matinee idols, used regularly on the most popular TV shows of the day: *Wednesday Night Fights* and *Friday Night Fights*. They were heroes in their hometown of Portland, Oregon. They had been in the gym from childhood, and their West Coast fans followed their lives and careers.

Denny had won and lost against a faded Sugar Ray Robinson and fought Carlos Monzon, Nino Benvenuti, Joe DeNucci, Ralph Dupas, Joey Giambra, Emile Griffith, Don Jordan, and countless leading names from the era. He held the world super-welterweight title between 1962 and 1963, capturing the vacant belt against Giambra before dropping it to Dupas.

Phil also defeated Robinson when "Sugar" was past his prime, and he boxed some of the big guns of the time, including Florentino Fernandez, Wilf Greaves, Don Jordan, and Terry Downes. They fought in an era when it was routine to box each month, when preparation for fights was either sparring or just more fights. Denny often boxed at least ten times a year. Phil's schedule was similar over a shorter span.

Brands like Gillette endorsed the TV shows, the entertainment was wholesome and competitive, and when you reflect now on the grainy black-and-white show reels of their fights, it was a different time at ringside. Spectators, wearing hats rather than snapbacks, produced thick clouds of cigar smoke that billowed through the roars of the crowd and cascaded over the ring. There were fifteen rounds in championship fights. There was only one world title in each of the eight weight classes. Yet there was no telling that life would turn black-and-white for the Moyers, trapped in lives of no color, observing decades of people coming and going from a nursing home with little understanding of what was happening around them and the memories of their wins over the greatest fighter of all time evaporated from even their own minds.

Denny eventually retired in 1975 but boxed twenty-two times in his final two professional years. Near the end, he had soaked up a ferocious beating from future middleweight champion Vito Antuofermo. Phil had retired ten years earlier, defeated in four of his final six fights. His last bout, in Boise, Indiana, saw him lose on points in a six-rounder to Jimmy Evans, who had won his only previous bout. That was in 1965 and Phil had not boxed for three years. He had been suspended in Oregon after suffering a detached retina against Downes in London. It was reported in the Eugene *Register-Guard* that Moyer fought under the alias Billy Bailey so he could get a license for his comeback.

In retirement, Phil became a boxing referee, and it seemed he had escaped with his faculties intact. That is often how it appears. You lose count of how many fighters who say, "I want to be able to retire in time so I can count my money" or "while I've still got my marbles." They think they will be okay.

"We didn't know at the time what the long-term effects of the sport were," said their seventy-one-year-old cousin, Tom Jr., a documentary producer who lives in Santa Barbara, California. "We didn't know about the long-term cumulative effects of head trauma and what it really was. We didn't know. Now we know today [and] we are opposed to the sport—while we understand that if someone wants to do it, it's their own right to work . . . it's their choice. But we are anti-boxing because of what happened to Denny and Phil."

Tom doesn't think the sport will end anytime soon, in part because it will always find a home. If one country bans it, another will have it. If one network won't broadcast it, another one will. Boxing will always find a way.

"[It is] the only sport in the world that rewards someone for giving the opponent a brain concussion," Tom said. "If it happens in soccer or football, you don't get away with that."

Tom's argument is compelling and persuasive, born out of decades of heartache. Denny and Phil were looked after by their father, their wives, their children, and their grandchildren. Over more than three decades, four generations of their family have had to live with the aftereffects of their boxing careers.

"It is really tragic," Tom said, shaking his head, before adding that the brothers did not believe their health had initially been compromised by boxing. "It started to manifest itself probably when they were in their forties and I don't think anybody became aware of it or what it was. They called it *punch-drunk*. They would say, 'Oh, he's punch-drunk.' And the guys in the gym would know other fighters who were punch-drunk, but they never thought it would happen to them. They really never knew what it was until we got modern science and you could actually look at the brain and you could say, 'These people have suffered multiple concussions over a period of time and it's impaired their ability to reason and understand what's happening and also their ability to physically move quickly, articulate words, and all of that.'"

Tom Jr. was part of fighting stock himself. Though he never boxed, his father, Tom Sr., "The Selwood Socker," was decent. His nine pro outings were all victories. He started fighting in Australia and finished his career in Portland, Oregon, as a National AAU champion who'd shared a ring with Sugar Ray Robinson in Buffalo in 1944. "He was really well regarded and a big deal back in the day," his son recalled. "Unfortunately, he quit. He just said, 'I'm, done, I'm not going to do this.' He had other opportunities and he never did show any manifestation of any kind of head injury from boxing. . . . [H]e was a smart guy and he said, 'There's no future in this.'"

Like his famous cousins, Tom, eight years younger than Denny, followed his dad to the boxing club—but as a spectator. "I was with my father, who promoted a lot of fights, and I was around the fighters a lot and the trainers, managers, and everything, but he didn't want me to pursue it."

Tom Sr. died in 2014. There were no CTE symptoms. It is the legacies of Denny and Phil that changed the family's attitude toward boxing.

"Why the civilized world allows it I will never really understand," Tom sighed. "The question is, why do we watch it? Why do people watch it? I would never let my grandson ever participate in boxing. And yet the irony of this is I believe it is a fact that the most superbly trained athletes on this earth are boxers. And they're in the most dangerous sport."

Tom Jr. used to watch Denny and Phil's fights on TV, and he recalled one particular bout Phil had with a horrid sense of dread: Phil's 1960 Madison Square Garden main event against Florentino Fernandez, the lead-fisted Cuban who smashed forty-three of fifty victims into premature defeats. Phil was dropped twice in round four and felled a final time in the fifth of a scheduled ten-rounder. "I remember the fight," Tom lamented. "Phil got hit and he got knocked down. He got up, lifted up his gloves, and he stumbled out to the middle of the ring and he finished the round, but for me as his cousin, watching it on TV, I didn't know [the damage that could have been caused]. . . . He was allowed to stumble into his opponent and to look at it . . . it just breaks my heart. It was on national television and we were all rooting for him. All of a sudden he got knocked down and we were saying, 'Oh, come on Phil, get up.' And now, knowing what we know and realizing what really happened to him, it's horrible. What happened was he got knocked down. He took a knee. He took a count to eight, stood up, he had no idea where he was, you could see it, and the ref held his hands up and said, 'Okay, go back and fight.'. . . [It] was just heartbreaking to see that. That's just traumatizing."

The referee was the distinguished Harry Kessler, but it was a different time then. Moyer was given every chance to fight on when he had no hope to turn things around. His only chance was to survive, but Fernandez was vicious and remorseless.

His team seemingly unperturbed, Phil was paired with Fernandez two years later but again he was knocked down on three occasions and stopped in round seven. At the center of it all was Phil's father, Harry, who had taken them to the gym, who had worked in their corners, and who had encouraged their every punch.

"Knowing it happened to his sons, how do you really live with that?" Tom questioned. "But he didn't know [the long-term dangers]. . . . Harry didn't know. Nobody did. We went into Harry's house one day and in his house in a closet was [Denny's] world-championship belt and he showed it to us and he said, 'You know, I don't think it was worth it. All I wanted them to do was just be amateurs and then these promoters get hold of them.' And you see what happens, these promoters are savages. They don't care one little bit about the safety of the fighters. They just don't."

In fact, Tom Jr. became a successful documentary producer because he believed it was his most powerful way of communicating his thoughts on the sport and the best way to share the experiences he and his family have gone through. He produced the film *After the Last Round* in 2010 hoping it would help people understand what happens in boxing.

"So what was the best way I could do it? It was to do a documentary about it," he said. "It weighed so heavy on my conscience, about what happened to my cousins, that I wanted people to know what the sport is about."

After the Last Round shows the disturbing footage of Harry nursing his boys, his nearing one hundred years of age with the siblings in their sixties and seventies. The documentary featured other fighters and other stories, but the Moyers are the sad spine of a narrative that stays with the viewer.

Some families have historically shied away from discussing having "punch-drunk" relatives. Tom thought it was an important issue to confront. "It helps raise awareness," he contended. "This is what happened to our family, and we didn't know any different. We just didn't know. It's the same thing I think with what's going on with mental health today. People used to hide the fact that they had a mental illness, whether it was, for example, depression, anxiety, or bipolar—whatever it was. They used to hide it and now people can draw attention to themselves and say, 'I suffer from a mental illness and I'm being treated for it and I'm not embarrassed about it because it's the same thing as if I had diabetes or if I needed glasses to see. I need help because my brain's just another organ that's ill, like a liver or a kidney.'"

Tom continued: "And I believe this, boxing is American football head injuries on steroids. . . . There's no question about it. There just isn't. You can't deny it. You can't spar a hundred rounds getting ready for a ten-round fight and not get hit in the head. And the sparring partners are nothing more than punching bags, you know? Everybody's talking about the dangers of football and a lot of people in America are saying they don't want their kids to play football. It's unthinkable that they would ever put their kid in boxing. Yet there's a culture of people that want to do it and for the life of me I don't understand why parents do it—and I think that it is child abuse. I'll say that. I think allowing your child to box is child abuse. They don't have the ability to reason [or] to understand. I don't think anyone should do it until they're about eighteen years old."

At eighteen Denny and Phil were setting out on successful pro careers, young fighters with dreams and ambitions to fulfill and a brutally tough era to navigate given the deep talent pools at welterweight and middleweight. The family witnessed their decline, from being supremely fit to incompetent. "It's hard," confessed Tom. "It's a long period of time to see someone go from the condition they were in into where they are now."

Denny and Phil Moyer sat in chairs from which they could not rise, in diapers they could not change, with ears that heard but could not listen and eyes that looked but could not focus. Their minds vaguely registered but did not retain. Phil was even unable to remember his wife, Mary Kay, although he was reassured by the presence of "that lady" when she visited.

"I don't think he was too sure of who I was," Mary Kay said in *After the Last Round.* "He's living over there [in the nursing home], but really he's dead."

Their daughter, Laura, recalled taking Phil to the nursing home.

"Please don't leave me here," he sobbed.

"I have to, Dad, it's for the best. We don't know how to take care of you any better," she countered.

"Just don't leave me here. Can I come and stay with you?" he begged, in one last effort.

"We can't do it."

And they could not. Not anymore.

Mary Kay said Phil had first become symptomatic in his fifties, perhaps even earlier.

It crept up on Denny's wife Sandy, too. "When it happens gradually, sometimes you don't notice it right away. He realized something was going on," she said.

Sandy also acknowledged that Denny needed round-the-clock professional care. "That was the saddest thing, because he thought he was coming home—and we knew he wasn't," she said forlornly.

One time, during a visit from Harry, he was sitting with his sons and talking about Denny when their father admitted, "He knows me but I have to remind him who I am."

"How have you been?" he asked Denny.

"Okay," came the mumbled reply. The former world champion was hardly able to talk and nonagenarian Harry was scarcely able to hear. As he shuffled down the hallway with Denny struggling to place one foot in front of another, Harry said optimistically, "You walk alright, do you do much walking?"

"Yeah," came the muted reply.

Nothing Harry said or did to assist his sons fixed anything. The brothers looked vacantly around while Harry searched for things to say that they might know the answer to. "What's the matter, Phil?" he asked, with the youngest fighting tremors. Phil, who later lost the ability to walk and was confined to a wheelchair, couldn't reply.

"I wonder if he's hurting," said Harry, concerned. He then stood, wiped the snot from Phil's nose and the saliva from around his mouth with a paper towel, and tucked it in his youngest son's lifeless hand. He sat there and watched them.

There is further footage of the Moyer boys bumbling around the nursing home grounds, clinging on to one another like human crutches. If one fell, the other would go too, which is why they were wearing helmets. It was a sorrowful and painful existence. There came a point when they could no longer recognize one another.

The hurt ended for Denny Moyer on June 30, 2010. He was seventy years old. The anguish of his father, Harry, ended on March 20, 2012. He had outlived his eldest son and was ninety-six.

For Phil, the sadness, the misery, and darkness remained. He lasted until January 15, 2014. Living death. Trapped in a corpse. He died aged seventy-five.

13
Labeled

"CTE SOUNDS A LOT BETTER THAN PUNCH-DRUNK"

The front line for fighters suffering neurologically might be the doctors trying to understand it, but there is a support system behind closed doors that has helped boxers more than scientists have. The wives of damaged former fighters have not just dealt with the athletes during scans, screenings, and medical appointments, they have monitored their loved ones around the clock. They have seen them deteriorate. They have been on the wrong end of mood swings. They have seen the depression and they have seen once-powerful men be humbled and impaired. With a sport that does not want to own its biggest problem, and scientists who do not have a full grip on what is happening or how to help, the wives of former boxers have been able to support each other during trying times.

Brenda Spinks, wife of former heavyweight champion Leon; Frankie Pryor, widow of light-welterweight Hall of Famer Aaron; and Rose Norton, widow of former heavyweight king Ken Norton have endured some tragically sad days. But by meeting at events like the International Boxing Hall of Fame induction weekends and staying in touch on the phone and through social media, they have been able to help one another cope with the challenges they faced as their iconic husbands transformed.

Aaron Pryor died in October 2016, aged sixty, having suffered from dementia. One of the greats, Pryor was a brilliant 140-pounder who lost just one of forty fights and was heralded for his two-bout rivalry with Nicaraguan legend Alexis Arguello.

"Even though they didn't know what to call it and they were saying to me, 'What's going on with your husband here?' they didn't have a word for it," Frankie Pryor said. "We all knew a long time before everybody else did that we're all dealing with the same thing . . . anger issues, possible addictions, nobody can manage their money, nobody can be left home alone, depression. . . . All of those things. We all started noticing that and I just happened to be one of the first wives in my circle that got the medical information, and I would pass it on, saying 'you need to get with this neurologist or ask for a certain type of doctor.' Then they started doing some of the studies. With what I know now, I know that Aaron was showing symptoms, a lot of symptoms, when I first met him in '91." Pryor would have been thirty-six.

Was she sure they were the symptoms of CTE? "I'm positive," she continued. "Because you know what? People look at an athlete and think, 'What were they thinking? Why did they behave in that way?' There's a loss of impulse control and all that, and there's a high correlation with drugs and alcohol, and I think that was all at play when I very first met Aaron."

"But back then there was no CTE," she said. It wasn't being discussed but then Pryor started to struggle with his sleep. Sometimes he would be up nonstop for two or three days and his temper was quick to boil as anxiety levels peaked.

Pryor had well-documented issues with drugs in the latter stages of his career. He and Frankie met in rehab but rebounded in life together, finally getting married and completing their nuptials in an emotional ceremony in 2003 at the International Boxing Hall of Fame. But Aaron's health continued to deteriorate and Frankie always felt it was because of the sport they had a mutual affection toward. "At the start, the neurologists knew it was boxing related," she said. "There was never a point where anybody thought it was anything else."

Aaron became religious and was ordained as a deacon in Cincinnati, but he never shook his troubles. Was it his poor socioeconomic background? Was it drugs and the toll they took on him? Was it the damage? And how terribly impairing if it was all three, which is what many fighters have to deal with? While Pryor struggled from one medical appointment to the next through his fifties, with Frankie by his side, he heard medical terminology he did not understand and could not or would not admit to. He was an all-time great. How could he be punch-drunk?

"Yeah," Frankie paused when asked to think about it. "He just couldn't really understand all that but he would be like, 'Oh yeah, I've got some memory loss. I've got some dementia from boxing. I'm an old boxer' and he would just laugh it off. But in terms of really understanding, you know, he didn't really understand it. He didn't. So I just took him to all of his appointments and made sure he got all the scans."

And unlike the scans that do not reveal the damage caused by the spread of tau protein, Pryor's scans actually did show that he had been injured in the ring. He had damaged his front temporal lobe, which could be detected via an X-ray. No autopsy was needed for that, even though, with the speed that Aaron declined at the end, the Pryors did not manage to leave "The Hawk's" brain behind for research. That remained a regret of Frankie's. Then, perhaps, more people would have talked about CTE, more people would have acknowledged it, and more research would have been done. Then, perhaps, it would not be the taboo subject in this, the hardest game.

Frankie believed it was not the toughness of the sport but the fragmented nature of the business that has prevented it being highlighted. With American football, everyone sued the NFL. In boxing, there are so many commissions and governing bodies, who do you go after? In a generation of blame culture, who do you point the finger at for allowing fighters to go on too long, to fight too often or too regularly?

"I guess because there's more centralized money in the NFL," said Frankie. "Boxing is such a loosely organized sport, it's not like there's one place you can go to register a complaint or ask something to be done. If I was to sue somebody, who would I possibly sue for what happened to Aaron? I would never do that, but I'm just saying that hypothetically. And who would want any sort of studies or to do anything? . . . [S]omeone asked my Aaron once, 'Oh gosh, Aaron, if you could do it all over again, I bet you wouldn't box, would you?' And he was like, 'What do you mean? Of course I'd box. Who would I be? I'm The Hawk.' I don't think athletes look at it the way we do. They cross that bridge when they come to it and if it happens, it happens."

And then it's too late.

"The Hawk's" son, Aaron Jr., became a professional fighter, winning twenty, losing eleven and drawing two. He was stopped three times and finally retired at the age of forty, by which time he had slipped into the sparring-partner mold. He had won just one of his last seven fights and had been a pro for thirteen years.

"I remember talking to Aaron Jr. one day," she explained. "I said, 'Don't you ever think about your dad? When you're training? When you're in a fight and doing all this?' And he would say, 'Well, you know Frankie, my case is different. I'm different from Dad.' And he has all these reasons [why] what happened to his dad couldn't possibly happen to him. He's like, 'You know, I didn't start boxing that early' or some-thing else. . . . And they're just really all made-up reasons, but he believes them. He really believes them. And in fact there's an Aaron Pryor the third [Aaron's grandson] that's in a boxing gym now. He's twelve."

The Pryor name is evolving, but in many ways the sport stays the same. However, acknowledgement from the wider sporting world means people are discussing it, even if it's not often boxing people. Awareness about this illness that is more than a hundred years old has started to spread in the house where it was conceived.

"I think now it's more acceptable to talk about [CTE], I've really noticed because we came out before Aaron died and it was out in the press that he had been diagnosed with it," Frankie continued. "But I started to notice that people would talk to me about that. Micky Ward was one. He talked to me about him being diagnosed and I think it's just more acceptable now, whereas fifteen, twenty years ago you just would never have said that. . . . I know that when Aaron was diagnosed, that term *punch-drunk*, nobody wanted that label. *CTE* sounds a lot better than *punch-drunk*. . . . I don't think that *CTE* carries that stigma the way *punch-drunk* did."

And she could be right. Look at the first medical journals. Not only did *punch-drunk* sound like a term of mockery, but the medical professionals who used it said that it happened to sparring partners, to journeymen, to fighters who were not that good. They said it did not happen to the better boxers, but they were wrong. Slick movers, punchers, warriors. . . . It does not discriminate.

Frankie has seen it, too. She has attended countless dinners, galas, events, and celebratory gatherings with some of the greatest fighters and has seen signs everywhere she looked. "Have you ever met a Hall of Fame guy, someone like Ray Leonard, Aaron, Hagler, Hearns? . . . You know that every single one of them is suffering with that. Duran. . . . When you really start talking to them, and now age is coming on, you can really see it. And I was in a position where, okay, maybe I'm not talking to a fighter about it, but the fighters' wives are coming to me because I have been pretty open about that. A lot of the wives would call me and say, 'Okay, what did you do? How did you cope? What kind of doctor were you dealing with?' Most neurologists are very, very familiar with CTE in today's world. Fifteen, twenty years ago, they were not."

Perhaps that is why countless fighters of the past died of what was labeled as Lou Gehrig's, Parkinson's, or Alzheimer's. Maybe it was CTE but they didn't have an autopsy and, if they did, the coroners might not have been looking for tau protein in the brain. Maybe the doctors of all of these old and rapidly aging fighters saw the symptoms of Alzheimer's and Parkinson's and diagnosed that. Maybe not. But the education is getting there even if the cure is nowhere to be found.

"They just know more about it now," Frankie added. "That's the thing. It's been studied so much that when you walk into a doctor's office . . . for example, take tremors. That's actually Parkinsonian Syndrome. They don't have Parkinson's. Like [Muhammad] Ali did not have Parkinson's. They said Parkinson's, his family and people around him. It's not Parkinson's. It's called Parkinsonian *syndrome*. So they can tell you all of those things and it makes you feel better and when a top-level athlete is getting it, it's not like it was before with the punch-drunk, you know? It's a different thing."

Yet Frankie does not think that boxing will take ownership of its own problem. Instead, she believes it will only be helped by other sports that do put more time, resources, and effort up against it. The lack of one overall federation puts a massive roadblock up to either making sure fighters do not sustain too much damage or that they are looked after if they do. "I really don't think that boxing is going to be the one to have a big impact on that," she said. "I think it's going to be the NFL and some-one with huge dollars. We know it's not going to be any promoter, right?" She laughed at the age-old stereotype that boxing has been pillaged by promoters, leaving arenas with their pockets stuffed with cash and a sea of broken bodies in their wake.

Ken Norton used to attend ex-boxer functions, along with his wife, Rose. "She went through an awful lot, too," Frankie went on. "People don't come out and just say, 'Oh, I've been diagnosed with this.' You have not met a fighter at the Hall of Fame, and I'm talking over the age of fifty, you have not met one that is not struggling with this. I do not know a former world champion who doesn't have CTE. I don't know one. And you've got to remember that you can go through years and years of just being at the early stages, and Aaron went through the early-to-middle stages for a very long time. Then, all of a sudden, it can just turn into late-stage stuff really quick, which was what happened to Aaron. What happened to Aaron essentially was that his brain could not send out any signals. So all of a sudden his heart's not working right, his lungs aren't working right, his kidneys aren't working right, so we were just dealing with medical issues all that time. And once that starts with the CTE, it's over. That's why he gained all that weight, because all of your major organs are just compromised. Everyone thought Aaron was gaining weight because he ate too much, that wasn't what it was. It's because their bodies can't keep up with all that when your brain is so damaged. That's generally what happened."

And then he was gone. At sixty. That great, colorful man who in retire-ment would still raise his right arm and bring a room to its feet by shout-ing "Hawk Time."

Frankie was fortunate to have a support group of other wives and widows. They developed a deep, practical understanding of the issues and then educated one another using experiences rather than data. They were not ashamed to talk about it. It was something only they knew and felt and something only they would understand.

There was another boxing widow they hoped would be part of their group. Frankie wished Lonnie Ali, Muhammad's wife, had publicly acknowledged the reason behind the icon's demise. Frankie felt that their involvement would have shone a light on CTE far faster and would have helped countless more fighters understand and admit to what had happened to them. If boxing could shut down the best—The Greatest—where is the shame in that?

"It was kind of always my one regret because the one fighter who had the notoriety and could have brought a lot of attention to this was Ali," Frankie concluded. "And then they went off on the Parkinson's thing and that really kind of, in boxing . . . I don't know if you've heard this said by any one of those top-level boxers, but that pissed off a lot of people in boxing that Ali's family chose to say, 'Oh, he has Parkinson's, it has nothing to do with boxing.' It has everything to do with boxing and no he didn't have Parkinson's [disease]. That was a shame. I don't think it was done maliciously. Maybe Lonnie didn't fully understand the impact, but just to say, 'It wasn't boxing, it was Parkinson's.' No it wasn't."

Frankie Pryor is a boxing widow. She lost her husband to the sport but there are no regrets that Aaron fought, and "The Hawk" would not have changed a thing. Do you have ten years at the top of life and struggle for forty, or live a mundane life forever without reaching the pinnacle of the mountain? Aaron made his choice and lived and died by it. Pryor's legacy in the sport is secure. He's in the International Boxing Hall of Fame and will remain one of the best to ever do it.

Although Frankie regrets that he did not leave his brain behind for research, she hoped Aaron's twenty years of neurological testing has left a different contribution to the sport. She is not the first lady of CTE but she, together with Rose Norton and Brenda Spinks, created a support system for one another and their warrior husbands that made their later lives more bearable.

14

A Warrior's Brain

THE COST OF A PRICELESS
LEGACY

"I have my days," Micky Ward groaned.

He leaned back in his chair, his eyes momentarily rolling as he was asked to describe his symptoms. Ward, from Lowell, Massachusetts, is one of boxing's modern-day gladiators. He took part in a succession of Fight of the Year candidates in his long career, often drawing the crowd to its feet by dropping his hands and swinging for the fences trying to out-tough an opponent.

His strategy frequently worked, but it came at a cost. The fifty-three-year-old does not slur his words. He does not shuffle when he walks. In fact, he can still turn in a decent 5K time. But he knows he has not come through the wars unscathed, and he has been told that, too. He was the straight-ahead gunslinger Harrison Martland, MacDonald Critchley, and the others warned would get damaged.

"There are some things like my memory," he said. "Long term I could tell you first-grade things I remember. I couldn't tell you yesterday, some things like that. Some things I can't really see, but my wife tells me. If I don't take my medicine, I get snappy. I get edgy and I didn't have that years ago. I'm very sharp-tempered if I don't take it. She will say to me, 'Did you take your medicine today?' and that's what I hate. If I've forgotten to take it and she can tell. And I'll snap, 'Yeah I took the medicine,' and then I'll go and take it."

He laughed at the lack of domestic bliss he inflicts upon his wife, Charlene, who has been by his side for almost two decades. She has seen a lot, including the bloodthirsty battles with Arturo Gatti that put an exclamation mark on his brutal career. But there were so many fights, so many stories, so many wars that the Gatti trilogy did not even get a mention in the movie of Micky's story, titled *The Fighter*, which is based on Ward's life and stars Mark Wahlberg in the lead role. The film saw Christian Bale score an Oscar for his portrayal of Ward's troubled brother, Dicky Eklund.

As Micky's exciting career wound down, Chris Nowinski approached him from the Concussion Legacy Foundation and Ward underwent physical and neurological tests with Dr. Robert Cantu in Boston in 2005. "He [Nowinski] knew I was a fighter, and he watched my fights and I believe he was a boxing fan. He's a great guy, a sports guy, played football at Harvard, he's a smart kid, he loves sport and he cares about people. And with me retiring from fighting and him probably knowing how many times I got hit, I guess he spoke to Dr. Cantu and said, 'Let's see if he has it [CTE symptoms].' I took numerous tests, a lot of them, and it came back that I do."

It is unlikely Ward will get better from here on out. The question is: how much worse will he become? "Now they can't tell how bad you have it until you're dead and then they can go inside and look at your head and your brain," Ward added. "That's why I've donated my brain and part of my spine, so they can look at the effects of concussion."

While he acknowledged the condition, he purposefully does not dwell on it. He is aware of what it may mean for Charlene and his daughter, Kasie. He knows it is something they will inevitably have to face together.

"No, I'm not scared," he snapped when asked. Then he paused and thought about it a little longer. "I'm not really joking about it, but I can't take it too seriously. So I am and I ain't. It is what it is. That's why I try to stay healthy, work out, and try to stay busy, because once you go off the deep end and you're doing drink and drugs, you know, it's going to get worse and—boom. I don't want to do that. I basically want to stay as I am."

Then he goes on a roller coaster of memories, of hard fights and sometimes harder sparring sessions. He thought nothing of punishing brawls, biting down on his mouthpiece, and fighting fire with fire. It's what he did, in the gym and in the prize ring. It's what secured his legacy in the hearts of a generation of fight fans. He symbolized a pure fighting integrity that cannot be coached, taught, or paid for.

But it is why he finds himself where he is today, and why he is arming himself with as much knowledge about CTE as he prepares for his future. You would think if he could do things differently he would, and perhaps the grueling training wars would be minimized.

He has his own theories now, but he didn't know any better back then. It was fight or spar regardless. Now he would not be so hasty. "Everybody's concussions are different," he continued. "Some people suffer from headaches. Some people suffer from depression. Some people get tired. Some people get angry. Some people want to hurt you. Some people want to hurt themselves. . . . Everybody's symptoms are different."

Ward admits he's boxed and trained while suffering with head injuries and probably concussions. "You're not going to say you can't spar," he tried to rationalize. "They're going to say, 'You're a pussy. You're this or you're that. Stop being a baby.' I would go and spar sometimes with the worst headaches but I was too proud. I didn't want to show pain or weakness. I was determined and I didn't want anyone to think any less of me."

What would he have done differently? "I think in the gym I would have mentioned it more," he confessed. "People ask me if I'd have fought any different. No. That was just me. The thing about it is there's no way they can stop concussions in boxing. The only thing you can do is probably minimize the sparring. I used to like to spar hard. You know what I mean? Because in my mind if I didn't get used to getting dazed then when you get hit in a fight—boom—you don't know what to do. I used not to like it but I wanted to get that zing because I would know how to react and I wouldn't be hurt. Some fighters, they pussyfoot around sparring and then they get hit in a fight and they're like, 'Whoa.'"

When asked why damage in the aftermath of boxing was not talked about much in the sport, he was unsure, but he thought it should be discussed. "It's real, it's happening," Ward said. "You can't deny it because it's proven with what it's done to fighters, to football players, to soccer players, to wrestlers. . . . People, because of money, want to turn the other cheek, but it's happening in sports right down to soccer where sometimes people are heading that ball at seventy miles per hour in the pros. But it starts with being a kid. What I believe, and I don't know this for sure, but three minors [head injuries] is a major. Just getting stunned in the gym with a right hand or whatever, not hurt, just stunned, that's a minor. I used to get those constantly. I don't know how many of those I had. Full-blown I had a whole bunch, but the minors are the ones that you don't think hurt but they still do damage. Then you're going back and sparring again. And again."

And again and again. Day in, day out. Fighters punch in at their office and they punch out. And then comes the fight. Boxers rarely enter the ring 100 percent, even though they are supposed to have trained for a peak. They may have suffered injuries or issues in camp, they may be going through personal problems away from the ring, they might have the flu, they could be weight drained. Anything. But they still do everything they can to hear the first bell. And when that sounds, they do everything they can to hear the final bell, unless they can get rid of someone beforehand.

Ward, whose blistering left hook to the body—rather than punches to the head—curtailed many a bout, was a tough man. Arguably too tough. In a two-part career, he went from prospect to gatekeeper. Then, after a layoff, he returned as a veteran and a contender. Regardless of what period you look at, he took a lot of abuse. He lost all seven rounds against Alfonso Sanchez before miraculously turning it around with a single body shot to finish the fight. Outweighed drastically by Mike Mungin, he somehow went the distance. Then, after violent seesaw battles with Shea Neary and Emanuel Augustus, he went to war three times with Gatti. Their first fight is often referred to as the best fight ever—in any era or weight class. Ward won that on points over ten rounds, but Gatti started the rematch sharply, caught Ward with a shot around his ear that caused him to pitch into the corner turnbuckle in round three, and that was all Ward recalled for the rest of the night but he boxed on for a further seven rounds—making it predictably brutal for Gatti, too.

"I don't really remember it," he said. "I just knew I was in a fight. I knew at the time I was in a fight but I can't really remember it. It was just instinct. Maybe that was because I'd sparred so hard, I was ready for it, and I was in such good shape that I was on autopilot."

Ward was not right for as long as two months after that fight, and then they fought a decider. Again it was ferocious. The two friends ripped into one another. Gatti broke his hand on Ward's hip. Ward floored Gatti with a huge right hand. After ten rounds and a few embraces in the ring post-fight, they wound up in beds next to one another in the hospital, laughing about their shared wars.

Ward did not box again following the third fight. Gatti did. Like Ward, Gatti was a thrill-seeker. His back catalog of highlight-reel fights was even longer than Ward's and as the Canadian's career wound down, Ward first became part of his entourage and then, for Gatti's final bout—a loss—his trainer. It was a storybook ending for them both and secured their already well-established legacies. Rather than going down in history individually, they went down together.

Gatti died under mysterious circumstances in Brazil in 2009 and Ward was devastated. They should have grown old together, done speaking engagements as a pair, gone on autograph signings as a double act. Now Ward goes to signings where half a picture will remain unmarked. But he still goes to events. His education when it comes to CTE means he no longer shrugs his shoulders when he sees a fighter struggling. He knows what's happening. "I see people at the Hall of Fame and I don't even know if they've even been diagnosed and some of them can't even speak a sentence, and I have it?" he asked rhetorically. "Maybe mine is different [from] theirs. I have some things that they have and they have other things that I don't have but you can't see. I don't have the speech but I have the headaches, the aggravation, and all the crap. Maybe they don't get that."

It doesn't sound too scientific, in typical Ward fashion, but it's accurate. He knows what he's talking about. Yet when Ward goes to fighter gatherings and is invited to premieres and events it's because people want to pay tribute to Micky Ward the warrior. As nice as Micky Ward the man might be, and as much as people appreciate him, it's the warrior they want.

And with that in mind, there is nothing he would change. Regardless of what lies ahead, he would not change what will define him. "That's just me," he said of his fighting style. "That's who I am. That's a priceless legacy to me. I fought the way I fought and I'd fight the same way again.

Honestly. God has a plan for me, I believe, and it was to fight that way, to meet my wife, and it's just his plan. I'm not a religious person but I do believe in Him, you know?"

Ward still works. Despite the big nights headlining on ESPN and on HBO, despite *The Fighter* ["Did it make you rich?" "I wish."], he gets up and works for relatives paving roads. He has always done it, even through his fighting career. There are no airs and graces about Micky Ward. There never have been, and that's another priceless quality that has endeared him to his fans. Ultimately, when he gets up and leaves home to go to work, his life has not changed and neither has he.

He's taking a break from training fighters in his Lowell gym because he's been burned out by the sport. He sees fighters churned out by boxing and left on the scrap heap. Forty years old. No qualifications because they focused on fighting. No plan B. Damaged.

He argued that there should be a union in boxing, where perhaps if fighters take part in a certain number of championship rounds, they get a pension for the rest of their lives. "The NFL has it, the NBA has it, MLB has it, NHL has it, boxing doesn't have it," he argued. "And when you're done with boxing, it's thank-you and—boom—the door closes. There's no pension plan for these guys and they put their lives on the line every time."

Ward himself is staying on top of his medical treatment because he's wary of what the future holds. "I go [to his neurologist] once every few months and they test me and I get medicine every month," he said. "[Wife] Charlene and [daughter] Kasie know I have it. Charlene knows when I'm good, when I'm bad, when I'm not taking it. She knows. She can tell by my voice. Anyone else . . . you, Dicky . . . no one else would notice. I've told Kasie about it and once in a while it will come up. I'm staying healthy, eating clean, and not drinking as much. . . . If you're out partying or you're soaking your brain with booze or whatever, I think that will make it worse. Or it could just get worse anyways. I don't know."

Some fighters have been reluctant to donate their brains to research, particularly the younger ones. Ward is not. Sincerity meets with dark humor when he speaks about it. "I hope it helps the next generation of fighters, not only in boxing but contact sports in general, and it helps them to understand better the effects of concussion," he said. "Really, I don't know what it can help but if it can help in any kind of way that's good."

Is it a big sacrifice? "No" he replied. "They're getting my brain. It will be like brand-new, never been used! I haven't used it in years." Ward chuckled but his eyes glazed softly and he went deep into thought. His future is uncertain, and he knows he has dependents that he might need to depend upon. Maybe in two years, maybe in twenty, but he hopes more boxers and their families will spearhead change and help sufferers while educating young boxers and trainers about steps they can take to improve their long-term chances. But this is boxing. It is an old sport with a closed mind. It does not benefit any of the governing or sanctioning bodies to work together, to give up their territory or share of any revenue, even if it could help fighters enormously.

"You know what?" Micky said, hand on his chin in consideration while turning his head left and right. "Boxing has been this way since day one and it's going to stay that way. Watch. It's sad."

15
Trapped

"I t hit the side and I felt a numbness and I remember falling and I could feel myself going down." In his next memory, Herol "Bomber" Graham was in the hospital being checked out. "After that, I watched it on television and it was then I really felt it. Watching it, I felt it."

Now, in a very different hospital several decades removed, Graham reviewed the fight and the punch on a mobile phone. He was in a north London psychiatric ward and round four against Julian Jackson began. Moments later, the shrieks of British boxing commentator Dave Brenner could be heard. "That's what we were worried about!"

The rerun was paused. Graham was lifeless on the canvas, having dropped suddenly.

Graham had spent eight months on a north London psych unit. It was not a fun place, but he was there because he was damaged. He was damaged from boxing. He did not slur his words, nor did he shuffle his feet. It even looked like he could go a few rounds now. In the not-too-distant past, he made an attempt at a marathon jump-rope world record. But he was told he had punch-drunk syndrome. It was, of course, a dated diagnosis meant to be consigned to medical history after J. A. Millspaugh's 1937 dementia pugilistica paper. But this was what Graham was told he had, and he was accepting of it, too.

"You do get punch-drunk," he said. "It does do that to you."

Graham's main problems were his short-term memory, or lack of one, and a biting depression that he could not shake. It drove him to multiple suicide attempts, which were the primary reason he was locked up. He could not be trusted. When he talked about suicide, there was a devilish grin that hinted he may just be a little out of control. Graham never felt the same after the Jackson thunderbolt, in or out of the ring. Even though the damage did not show early, it manifested itself, along with thirty years of fighting, and resulted in his condition today. "When I went back in the ring [after Jackson], I felt that I wasn't all there," he said. "There was the apprehension of, 'Shit, is it going to happen again?' That's in your head, that you don't want it to happen again, but you just think it and think it. But I wasn't the same because that was in my head."

At the time, he believed he could carry on his fine career at a decent level. All he had to do was hit, move, and not get hit like that again.

But Graham was by now running on fumes, and soon the time came to call it quits that resulted in a dark feeling that had gnawed at him for years. "Of course, when you walk away it's hard," he admitted. "But my depression was way, way in front of that. It must have been five, six years prior to that."

There were issues away from the ring, including heartbreak, a fallout with trainer Brendan Ingle, abuse he'd suffered as a child, and more besides. That went with him into the ring, and crushing losses did not help. Neither did the constant references to him as the best British fighter to never win a world title. What kind of honor is that? That neither puts money in the bank or a belt on the mantelpiece—and it certainly didn't open any lucrative doors.

Then the alcohol came. "I did drink [before], but not to that extent," he said. "I know that drink and alcohol is a killer. I did have a drink and more so after boxing. It nearly became a problem because as the depression kicked in I was looking for a shield, the shield was alcohol, and I just went overboard with it. I was on medication as well and that's how

I ended up here because this is my third time [in the ward]. The first time was after the boxing."

Graham looked deceptively fit and well, yet said he only managed the odd powerwalk. He wanted to do more, but the depression chains him to chairs and he sits and festers and cries. "Being in here is like being in a prison, but I've never been in a prison, of course," he continued. "But you are locked up. I have leave so it's not as bad, but sometimes with the depression, it's escorted leave only, so they will be watching over me all the time. Wherever you go, they go with you."

Graham actually has been to prison, just not as an inmate. He practiced his moves in prison, under Ingle's watchful eye. The wise old trainer would put Graham in jails, in working-men's social clubs, and he even took them to nightclubs where he let anyone interested try and hit his boys. His boxers were not allowed to punch back. On Saturdays and Sundays, they got out of the gym and tried to avoid being struck in the head.

"There was some bloody horrible places we went to but it was good fun," Graham recalled. "You look at them and some of them were huge and looked tough with skinheads or whatever, but I thought the people wouldn't touch me."

He continued: "The rules were they could touch me anywhere above my waist so all I did was put my hands down and moved around. But I had to be careful because in prison, they will just go out to smash you. They don't care. If they can do some damage to you, they will, and I couldn't let that happen. They were going for the face as well—it was open sparring and I'd move out of the way, grab their hands, and move their hands round so it would spin them round and they'd get frustrated. When they got frustrated that was it, finished, I had them where I wanted them.

"Sometimes there were women doing it and I remember I was moving away and—bam—she hit me with a backhand. There's always one. Under a photograph in the paper it said, 'The only person to hit Bomber Graham,' and it was this woman. No one ever hit me full on. If they did, I would have gone in for them. . . ." He laughed heartily, again a mischievous smile crossing his lips.

"In the nightclubs there were some big boys, there were fighters in there, and they'd come out to destroy you. We had to be on our best behavior and on our best form, otherwise you'd get caught. They'd [announce where we were going] on the radio, they would say 'Bomber Graham will be at Pine Grove Country Club,' that sort of thing, and we did it all over Sheffield. Sheffield's quite big. And sometimes the places were packed and Brendan would say, 'Herol, don't get hit. But don't go too hard on them.' They could hit me but I couldn't go hard on them, and it was good for my boxing. They were good days."

The Sheffield "Bomber" was a slick and quick mover. He owned a jerky style and was nearly impossible to hit. There is more than one story of a top sparring partner throwing down his gloves unable to strike anything and storming from the ring.

And those memories, in his long-term memory bank, still linger. He can recall his first day in the Ingle gym more than forty years ago in great detail. "It was a Sunday morning," he reflected. "This is what I mean . . . you see how my brain goes. All those years ago and I remember it was one Sunday morning. I'm going to start crying again . . . I went to Brendan's house [he recalled both his and Brendan's postal addresses from the time], he lived at the bottom right-hand side of the road. I went to his house, had a hot drink, and we went to the gym. I remember looking at everyone and thinking, 'Oh, I wonder what they're like?' He introduced me and said I was going to do some sparring, told me to get my gear on. There was a guy there, Mick 'The Bomb' Mills, and he threw some heavy shots, and there was some other guy, Robert Wakefield, and Brendan said, 'You have to move with them.' At the end Mick says, 'Fuck me, I can't fucking hit him.' I was just moving, moving out the way. And he was shouting, 'Stand still you bastard!'"

"Listen," Graham said tearfully. "I can remember all these things from back in those days."

Those days have gone, slipped away, replaced by a barren nothingness, an existence where fame, skill, and being the best British fighter never to win a world title counts for nothing. Graham paused to look around at the ward's brick walls. "It's no life," he said. "But when I think about it, I sometimes think, actually, it's the best place for me in a sense that the medication . . ." he tailed off, talking about his access to therapists and antidepressants.

One wondered if he was not becoming institutionalized. Even though he seemed so different from the people around him he felt he belonged there. Asked whether he believed he could cope in a halfway house, a stepping-stone back into society, he sighed. "I was anxious to get out, but what's going to happen? Will I be okay?

He paused and looked around at the eccentric cast of supporting characters around him. Some gave the impression of being on the edge; others were lost, staring into parallel universes. Graham allowed himself a moment to believe he was not one of them. "I hope they don't get out before me," he said. He nodded toward a resident. "That one, I feel for him. He can't communicate with anyone. He doesn't know what he's doing."

Yet Graham was on friendly terms with some. He nodded at one, winked at another, high-fived and cracked jokes with others. Granted, his one-liners were either not understood or left unappreciated, but he backed them up with a winning smile every time. "What's the use in not making friends with people," he said. "Or else you're looking over your shoulder all the time. I know why. It's a self-defense thing for me. I could flip at any time, but I don't really get aggressive. I can talk my way out of a fight in here."

His popularity earned him a job offer on the ward, helping the staff. He considered it but rejected the opportunity. He admitted the proposal had its benefits, though. "At least I'm here. At least if I get depressed or anything happens to me, I'm here already," he smiled.

Graham was asked to think back to his youth. Was he aware of the possible long-term damage of boxing? "No. No chance," he answered emphatically, shaking his head. "'Oh it won't happen to me.' Don't be so stupid. It's like me—look how many boxers don't box my style and don't jab and move, jab and move. They'd rather go forward and take the fight to them and they don't bob and weave, they're just going forward and getting smashed in the head and it's the impact of the glove onto the head, it shakes the head back and forward. Then the brain is shaking all the time. I would say to them, I would tell them what could happen. 'Be prepared—you can get brain damage.'"

"They're going to have to do something," he continued, while touching on the CTE discussions being had in rugby and soccer. "They have to do something because boxing is dangerous, end of story. They all know that. The adults know it. The kids don't. I think they will do it where they can't hit the head and it will be body sparring. It will be unpopular but what do they do? Ban the boxing? And they can't because then it would go underground. There's someone in here, he's around twenty-five, and he's punch-drunk from bare-knuckle boxing. Personally, I think it should be banned. Medically it's trauma to the brain and it can kill you. You say, 'Okay, I know it can kill me but I still want to do it.' Okay then. Fine. Then do it. But let them know what can happen and then it's their choice or the parents' choice. But you've got to let them know. If you hide [the risks], you become a criminal. If I'm not telling you [about the risks] and I'm your manager, the onus is on me. Not them."

Graham then started hypothesizing about different safety measures. It was clearly something he had thought about over the years. He thought headgear made things worse. He believed a lot of damage was done in the amateur years, when fighters were still young. He said body sparring wouldn't help come fight night. He wondered whether there should be an age limit "because the longer you do it, the worse you're going to get."

Graham thought it boiled down to getting youngsters to learn the art of hitting and not getting hit, teaching head movement to avoid punches. But that is what he did. He was one of the most elusive fighters of a generation. Yet he believed defense plus education about long-term damage was the way forward.

"The more they know about it the better they will protect themselves in the sense that they won't get it [damaged], they won't go in for the fighting or they won't do the boxing," he said. "What do they want to go in and get beat up for? As I've always said, 'He who runs away lives to fight another day.' I say, 'Go in there and don't get hit.' Smash him as much as you can, hit him, because that's what he's going to do to you. Hit him and don't get hit,' but they want a tear-up."

Asked how many times he was hit in the head, Graham, who won forty-eight of fifty-four fights, responded, "I'd say . . . not as much as a lot of them, but it's enough in the sense it's hurt me and I've got brain damage."

Those who tend to him on the ward try to find a balance for him, using drugs to calm his explosive outbursts without sending him into another realm.

He also discussed what happened to him with doctors, though they seem to be behind the times. Even calling it "punch-drunk syndrome" makes one wonder how much the doctors knew about CTE and what *was* actually happening to Graham. "I've had the EEG scans and they said from the first one I had to the second one nothing has changed and they're pleased with that because they say as your age goes on, your loss of memory increases."

"The comfort is that through the fighting, I had a good time. I had the bad fight there [against Jackson], but who in boxing doesn't have a bad fight?" he continued. "You have the expectation that you're going to get hit. You don't think someone's going to throw a bomb at you, but it does happen. I've seen worse things than that happen in the ring. I've seen younger kids and older people get smashed up. I wouldn't want that. I'd rather a clean shot, gone, and then you come to life and think, 'Oh, I'm not dead actually. I'm still alive.'

"I know people who haven't boxed and they have the deterioration without boxing. I'm fifty-nine this year. I'm a good fifty-nine. Sometimes I have to write things down and it jolts my memory and then it gets working. The stuff at the back of my head is still there. At the front of it . . . it's not there."

He reverted once more to educating fighters and trainers about the hazards of boxing. He himself had managed to fall between gaps. He reckoned that his trainers had not warned him Jackson was a puncher, when he was one of the hardest hitters the game had seen. And that fight only happened in Spain because the British Boxing Board of Control would not license Graham over concerns surrounding his health, specifically his eyesight. He had suffered a detached retina and faced the prospect of losing his vision altogether if he fought on.

But CTE was not in boxing parlance, and Graham boxed in a simpler time when it had not been accepted that it would happen to "runners." The Sheffield star had not been told what might happen long after the cheering stopped and the audiences filed out of the arena.

It is too late for Graham, who now lives with demons and regrets. He said he "can't be bothered" to watch tapes of his fights, even the glory nights, and he lived with the remorse that he never listened to one piece of advice over anyone else's: his own, "because he who runs away lives to fight another day and it hurts me because that's what I say to everyone, 'Run, run, run.' And I didn't. If you're running away and hitting him, he's missing you. And I didn't do it for Julian Jackson and it chews me up. He had been brilliantly outboxing the feared "Hawk," then the lights went out and everything changed.

"Sometimes I think I wouldn't be here if I'd beaten Julian Jackson. If only . . . if only. But it's always if only. They're small words 'if only,' but they mean something big, although they can't help."

Graham has hopes for the future without having them raised. A group of like-minded and kind boxing people in the United Kingdom have assembled a conglomerate and hope to build a retirement home for former fighters. Ringside Rest and Care has applied for charity status to benefit "countless boxing personnel who find themselves suffering from depression, alcohol dependency, injuries and illness attributed to boxing." The dream is to create a thirty-six-bed home with medical help and facilities for former boxers to receive long- and short-term care. It is thought to be able to run at a cost of £1.5 million per year.

"We should do that halfway house, for the boxers who have been injured where they can have the medical treatment," Graham said optimistically of the ambitious project he hoped to become a beneficiary of. "If they do that it would be swathe, a cool place. It's going to be plush. How many boxers are there in my condition or worse and it will help them? Somewhere to wind down for the boxers themselves."

Those backing the home have talked of a cinema room where boxers can watch their old bouts. But some might argue that having fighters living in the past is not a way to help them cope with the future. Rather, the home should include workshops, educational options, and plans to help them with life after the final bell, whether it's elocution lessons, fitness classes, or anything else. Some of the residents could be as young as forty. They can't spend another forty years looking back on a few memorable nights. They have to have structure and a strategy to move forward.

But the idea of a care home for CTE patients, a place where fighters can understand what is happening to them and a place where families will be able to get help, is certainly better than what Graham has today.

The boxing fraternity is a supposedly tight-knit network that looks after their own. Graham seemed abandoned.

"Do you feel like you get any support?"

"Two minutes," he pleaded, excusing himself. He returned waving a card from the Essex Ex-Boxers Association (EBA), and he seemed generally thrilled to be remembered. Members wishing him well had signed it. "I got that today," he said. Then, with utter sincerity, from a sport with multimillion pay-per-views, global superstars, and a huge international fan base, he looked genuinely delighted, happy in the knowledge that a handful of people outside the walls had thought of him.

"They keep in touch, which is good of them," he smiled, staring proudly at the names of those who were sending him good wishes.

He was perhaps the best boxer never to win a world title. One of the most skillful to ever do it, yet all he had to show for it was a dizzied, sad mind and a greeting card thanking him for his efforts and hoping that he would get well soon.

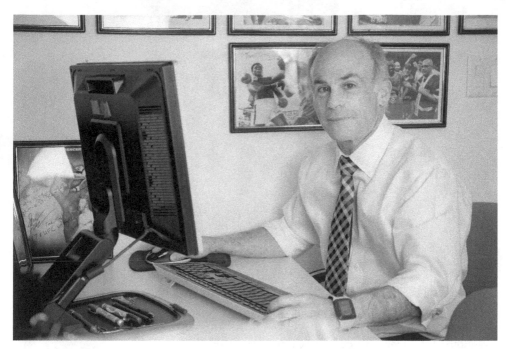

Dr. Charles Bernick leads the Professional Fighters Brain Health Study in Las Vegas. *University of Nevada, Las Vegas*

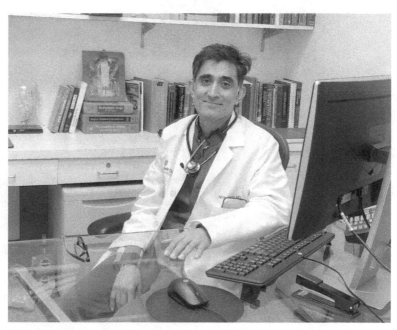

Ringside physician and neurologist Dr. Nitin Sethi pictured in his office in New York City.

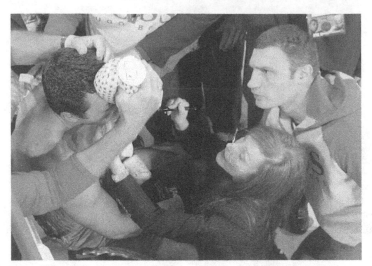

Dr. Margaret Goodman assesses Wladimir Klitshcko. Now she tries to make sure boxing is a clean sport by running the Voluntary Anti-Doping Association. *Getty Images*

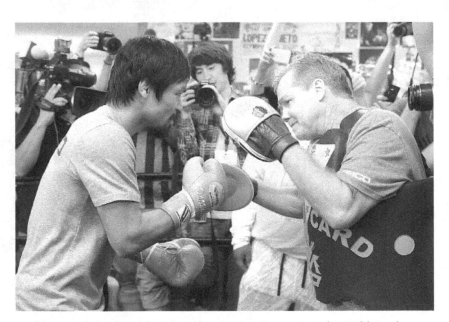

Freddie Roach works with star student Manny Pacquaio in his Wild Card Boxing Club. A former crowd-pleasing fighter, Roach has had Parkinson's for more than thirty years. *Getty Images*

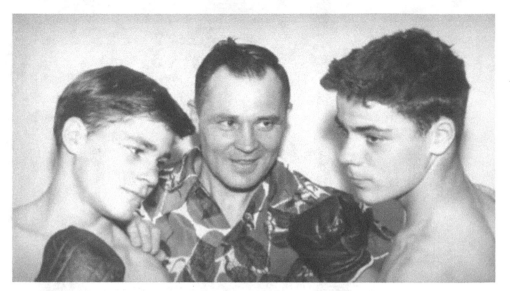

Phil Moyer (left) and Denny (right) pictured with father Harry were excellent fighters. Both were okay when they retired, but their health faltered and they spent decades in a rest home and had to wear helmets in case they fell.
Tom Moyer, After the Last Round *documentary*

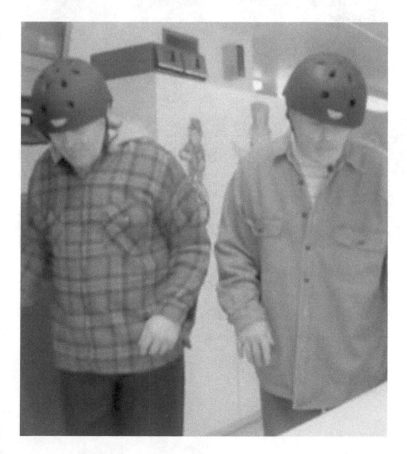

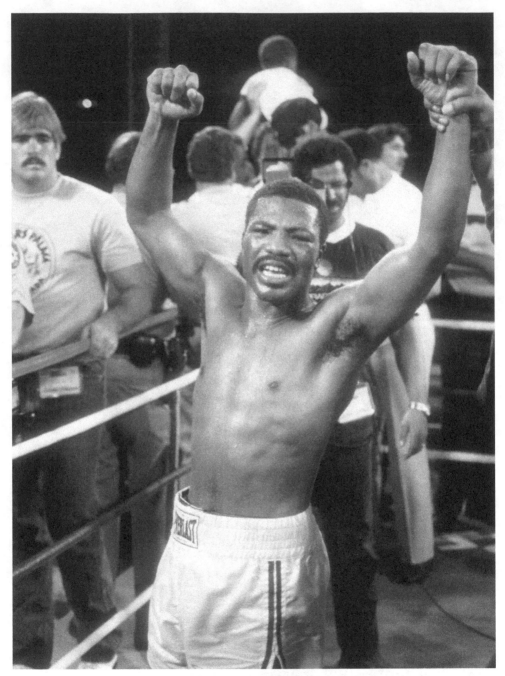

Aaron "The Hawk" Pryor was one of the all-time greats. *Boxing News*

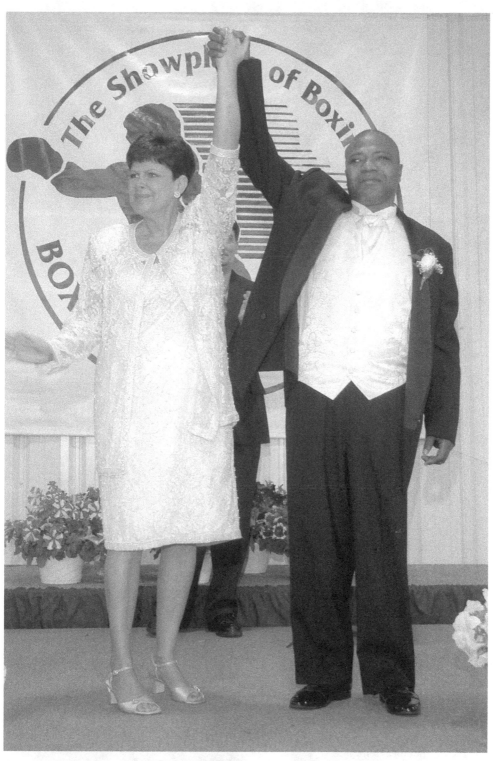

Aaron and Frankie tie the knot at the International Boxing Hall of Fame in Canastota.
International Boxing Hall of Fame

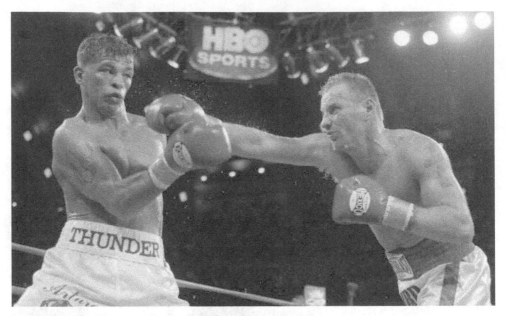

Micky Ward and Arturo Gatti waged a historic war but, in retirement, the ever-popular Ward has struggled with mood swings and short-term memory loss. *Getty Images*

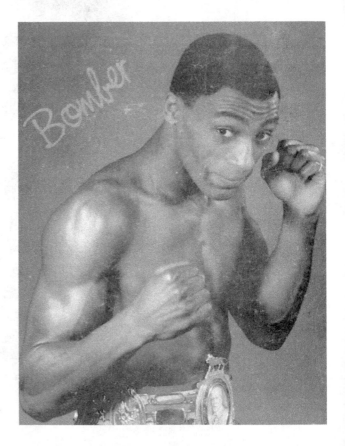

Herol "Bomber" Graham strikes a pose in his prime. *Boxing News*

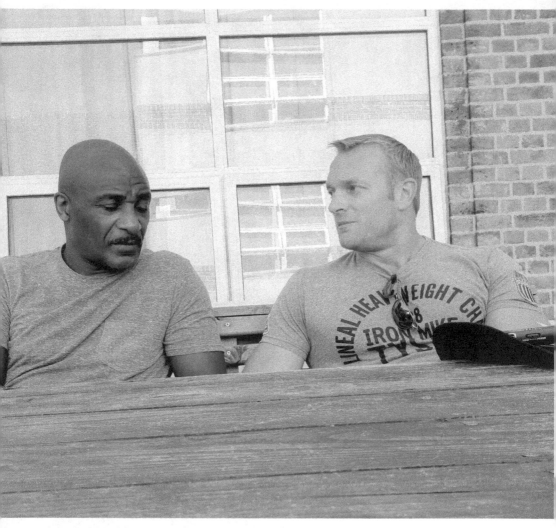

Herol Graham and the author meet in a psychiatric ward in London.

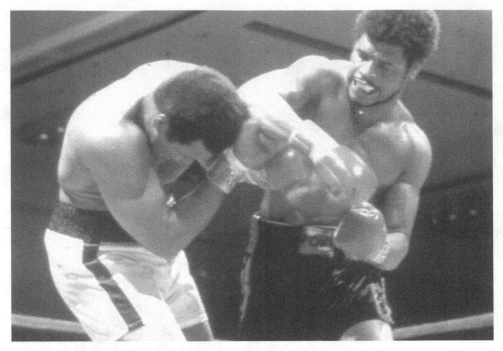

Leon Spinks storms forward against Muhammad Ali in their first fight. Spinks won Olympic gold and the world heavyweight title and is pictured below with his wife, Brenda, at their home in Las Vegas in 2019. *Boxing Hall of Fame*

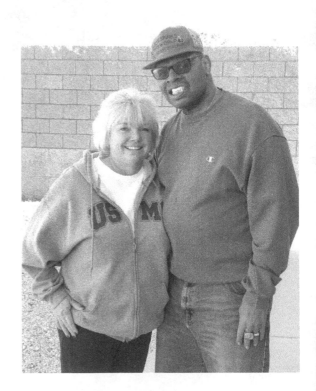

16
Risk Takers

DO FIGHTERS RECOGNIZE
WHAT'S AT STAKE?

"I'm on the back end, I know what it's like," said former WBO heavyweight champion Shannon Briggs.

The big New Yorker was still fighting as he neared his fiftieth birthday. He called out the big names and wanted the big nights even though he fought George Foreman and Lennox Lewis more than two decades ago. He knows something is wrong with him and feels he will struggle in time.

"So many brothers and sisters around the world are suffering from head trauma in contact sports, and I'm always confident there's a cure around the corner, that they're going to cure it in the next couple of weeks," he said, "I know I've got something wrong with me, I know all these punches are going to eventually catch up to me, so I'm reading about CTE and I started taking CBD and I haven't had a drink in seven years. I poured the [antidepressant] pills down the toilet the day I tried cannabis, I hadn't smoked since I was a kid, I was asthmatic all my life."

"It's a very real thing, isn't it?" said former IBF cruiserweight world champion Glenn McCrory about long-term damage, before adding, "but if you're in the game of boxing you're going to have the ramifications in later life so it kind of gets pushed away. It's never something I thought would come back to me. When you're boxing you never dwell on anyone getting injured, you never dwell on anyone going into a coma or getting killed. I remember staying up and listening to Johnny Owen [who was killed following a bout with Lupe Pintor in 1980] on the radio. It didn't stop me, put me off, or make me think anything different."

McCrory had thirty-nine pro fights in a nine-year career and served as a sparring partner to a prime Mike Tyson. He worries about his memory and thinks the responsibility of education about the real risks, long- and short-term, lie with the managers and trainers.

"It's really important to be able to pull a kid to one side and say, 'You know what? Get a day job or do something else,'" he said. "Obviously that's very important, but it doesn't happen because managers and trainers just think of the next payday and the next kid on the block. If the people around Ali could let him go into the Berbick fight, and if you watch him go into that fight now, you can see he's got Parkinson's and you think, 'How did the world let that happen?' But Ali had always said he wouldn't change the first bit of his life for what happened in the second bit."

McCrory suffered with demons away from the ring, as did middle-weight contender Matthew Macklin, who fell short of world-title glory against Gennady Golovkin, Felix Sturm, and Sergio Martinez. Macklin is not sold that boxers struggle because of head injuries, and he understands the sport and the fighters well. "Depression, alcoholism, retirement, there's a lot of things that overlap there so it's difficult to say it's because of the head trauma," he said. "There are obvious things with repeated head trauma, but, being retired at thirty-odd years of age, I know people who struggle when they retire at sixty-five because they've been doing something every day. A man has to have purpose in life and I suppose when you're sixty-five, you've got kids, you've got grandkids, you're slowing down, you're happy to chill out and they're your purpose. But when you're thirty, thirty-five and you've been a very fit and active sportsperson, it's like, 'Well, what am I going to do for the rest of my life?' And most of the time they haven't thought that far ahead. They know they can't box forever, but they don't really put many plans forward for what they're going to do. And I think it's impossible to appreciate how it's going to feel. It's difficult, and the first couple of years, I thought I knew what it was going to be like, but it was tougher than I thought—even being busy. I probably hadn't stopped to process it. I don't think I took enough time to reflect on my own career."

But Macklin has seen fighters he came through with start to deteriorate. Welterweight David Walker, a TV darling in the 2000s in the United Kingdom; Howard Clarke, a journeyman who wound up on the receiving end of Fernando Vargas in New York; and Mancunian star Michael Gomez, for instance, who has been diagnosed with dementia pugilistica.

"I knew I wasn't the same fighter at the end of my career, I knew I didn't want to do it anymore if I'm honest, but I was clinging on because you've worked hard your whole career and suddenly you're in a position where you can earn good money because of your name and you're still in that world top bunch and you think if you get the right break, you can get a shot. But I've been in a lot of hard fights and I sparred hard, I [got] cut and bruised up and had a lazy right eye that I was born with and I've had a lot of trauma on the left side, and if I was to lose sight on that side or suffer a detached retina. . . ."

He paused for thought. "When you're young, you're fearless. I was just reckless and hungry, but, as you get older, you think about it. One of my favorite fighters is James Toney [and] he's struggling to string a sentence together. I was training in the Wild Card back in 2010 and 'Terrible' Terry Norris—what a great fighter he was—he could barely talk. And it's not just the fights and the KOs. Some of these fighters are half-concussed and then they box a week later, then the same thing again, so they didn't get knocked out and get twenty-eight days [suspension], but they still took a lot of damage. And we don't know what effect that's having and it's a lot of that trauma that isn't taken into account."

When asked about whether fighters are hurt by the terminologies *punch-drunk syndrome* and *dementia pugilistica,* Macklin said the name was irrelevant. "You can throw in as many euphemisms as you want, you've been banged around the head and suffered trauma over the years and it's a form of brain damage," he explained. "I was definitely aware of it. I don't really think about it too much. I feel good but I know it's progressive and it can kick in at any time. I feel good today. I haven't fought in two years. I had a lot of hard fights and hard spars but I had periods of inactivity too. . . ." Macklin continued: "I think it's an acceptable risk if you're a Formula 1 driver, or you're a horse rider, do you know what I mean? Anything like that. I just don't think people think that far [long-term] ahead. People think about now. People do things in spite of relatively short-term risks and they think, 'I will cross that bridge when the time comes but right now I'm going to spar, or I'm going to be world champion.' People don't think about it until it happens and then they may say, 'I wish I hadn't done this' or 'I wish I hadn't done that,' but I think that's life."

Critics have long targeted Amir Khan, who won a silver medal at the 2004 Olympics and then captured world titles in the pros, because of his chin. The criticism had been that he had no punch resistance, but as he entered his thirties, he had been through wars with Marcos Maidana, Willie Limond, Samuel Vargas, and countless others. He had been harshly knocked out by Danny Garcia, Breidis Prescott, and Saul Alvarez, and he had been in competitive spars for more than a decade. The teenage sensation from Athens had high mileage.

"There is a lot of long-term damage in boxing," Khan said. "Look, you're getting punched in the head for a living and you're getting a lot of damage to the head—the brain and the body. It's important you do your medicals often, that you meet the right doctors, that if you've got headaches or whatever, you need to get checkups. There's no point saying, 'Ah, it will cost me,' because in the long-term it will cost you a lot more. I like to keep myself fresh and I'm lucky that when I've been knocked out, it's been that one shot that's knocked me out instead of taking numerous big punches. I'd rather be knocked out with one big punch than be hurt and take many more. Probably the biggest damage I took in a fight was with Maidana because I stood there and showed too much heart, and I took big shots but I gave big shots back. Those are the fights that can give you big problems in the future. You don't want too many of them. It's all about being smart. I don't like being hit. I like to move my head a little more and that helps me keep out of trouble."

Khan admitted he cannot remember much of the Maidana fight and acknowledged that he had been to war in gyms throughout his time in boxing. One acid test came after he rebounded from the Prescott destruction under his new trainer at the time, Freddie Roach. He was put in with Manny Pacquiao, then arguably the most ferocious knockout machine in the sport. They battled it out, supposedly on even terms. And while Khan's confidence began to return, the mileage would have accumulated.

"Sparring is something you need to do, but I am very wary about what you should and shouldn't do, and if you are taking any damage or big headshots, you need to go to the doctors," Amir insisted. As Khan recovered from his big KO loss to Canelo Alvarez, he went into the jungle as part of the cast in *I'm a Celebrity . . . Get Me Out of Here!* He needed the break. While in the jungle, Khan was asked by another celebrity when his daughter's birthday was. He could not recall it but insisted his memory always was haywire and it's been no worse for boxing.

"I forget things," he said, when asked about the show. "That's normal for me. I've always been like that. I don't think it's anything to do with boxing." Then, ironically and accidentally playing into the stereotypes being discussed, he joked, "It was probably from when my mum slapped me around the head as a youngster."

While Khan's jesting puts a lighthearted spin on a hard-to-discuss subject, he knows that people avoid the topic of damage. "People are scared to talk about it, and I think it should be addressed. People need to talk about it and get help. I'll be honest with you, there's a lot of times I forget things and you shouldn't be scared of telling people because there should be somewhere we can get some help. I still feel sharp-minded but I still get my checkups done, that's something I will always do."

Former heavyweight contender Bert Cooper was in his share of slugfests through the 1990s. Yes, he sat out a few when the going got tough, but he was in wild shoot-outs with Evander Holyfield, Ray Mercer, and Michael Moorer, among many others. He was also a warhorse in the gym. He was a paid-for sparring partner, a hired hand to go rounds with the champions who were sharpening their tools for upcoming title fights. His memory was not so sharp, he'd battled addictions to drink and drugs and struggled with depression.

"I have early-part dementia," Cooper said. "I was diagnosed in Vegas by neurologists. Sometimes I get tripped up on my words, I can't think, and my equilibrium is off a little bit."

Was he worried about it worsening? "Nah. My grandma lived to a hundred, my dad to eighty-six when he passed of cancer a couple of years ago. I don't drink or smoke. . . ." It's a fighter's outlook. You play with the cards you are dealt.

"You don't think about it, you just go ahead and do it. People don't like to talk about it but it's nothing to be embarrassed about. I don't mind talking about it. I would make that sacrifice again and I did make that sacrifice."

While Cooper, who died at the age of fifty-three of pancreatic cancer in May 2019, was plying his particularly belligerent and brutal trade, Christy Martin was rising to prominence as the world's premier female fighter. She was on Mike Tyson undercards, on the cover of *Sports Illustrated,* and something of a media darling. Now fifty-one years old, she's not symptomatic but is aware that could change, though she's not sure it would be addressed as people won't discuss it.

"Absolutely it has been a taboo subject," she agreed. "It's just not talked about. The real dangers and risks are long-term, punches and the punishment we've taken to our heads."

Typically, like all fighters, her mindset is "bring it on" if the disease wants to fight her. And when you have a story like hers, poor health is something that doesn't frighten you as much as it should. This was someone who survived getting stabbed three times, shot, and was then left for dead by her deranged ex-husband.

"Personally, no," she said, explaining why she doesn't fear it. "I've already been through hell, and I think God has a bigger plan for me." She continued: "It's taboo because there's no way that we can't be brain injured in what we do. God did not create us to be punched in the head and our brains to have this much trauma. It's taboo because if we talk about it, then boxing's going to go away, so we can't hurt our sport by talking about the possibilities of what the future holds."

Then, with that familiar warrior's refrain, she continued, "I wouldn't change anything. That's who I am. I would never have chosen boxing as a sport to follow had that not been my style. My character and who I am is not to go out there and be the pretty boxer; my personality and my character is to go out there and get into a war and that's when I was at my best, when I could get somebody to go into that war with me. And I'm proud of that."

But it's the kids and those at the start of the journey who dream of holding world titles above their heads and retiring on a mattress full of money, with fleets of exotic cars in their garages and jewelry boxes full of watches who do not consider the possibility of winding up unable to look after themselves.

Anthony Fowler was a touted amateur who fought at the Rio Olympics in 2016. Now a pro prospect, with a physical, all-action style, he spoke of his career options a few months before he lost his unbeaten record. "Obviously I know getting punched isn't good for me, but I've got nothing else to do with my life," said the Liverpool hope. "I'm a boxer. I am what I am, so hopefully I will get my money and get out with my wits intact."

He's been in the sport a while already—even though his pro journey is nearer the start than the end—and said he has witnessed fighters damaged by their time in the ring. "I've seen a bit of both," he added. "Some of them have come out with money, some of them have come out well. Look at someone like Carl Froch, who I always compare myself to. He's got his wits about him. He was in some tough, tough battles and he's doing well now so hopefully I can do the same."

There is an awful lot of hoping for the best in this sport, but at no point is getting hit in the head beneficial.

"I've been getting punched in the head now for twenty-plus years," said former world super-middleweight champion George Groves, Froch's bitter rival. "I would be shocked if that doesn't have a negative effect on my health in years to come. It's going to be very sad if I get dementia one day, but I like to say I wouldn't be surprised but I might not remember. It's risk–reward. You pick a job and it could have a negative effect on your quality of life, but you hope you have already lived your life by the time those negative effects kick in. . . . If you get as much out of boxing as I have, I'm pretty sure you'd trade that off for the risks that are involved. But at the same time, once you've got a family, you start thinking past boxing and you're thinking, how far are you willing to push it? I don't want to be on a kidney waiting list because I've been making weight for twenty years, or I don't want to be on long-term medication for Parkinson's because I've taken one too many punches."

Groves's openness was unsurprising given his nature to address awkward subjects and his cerebral approach to his career and life. He would not have turned a blind eye at the ex-boxers meetings where he has seen weathered fighters left decrepit and wandering that familiar avenue of sadness.

"Once you're boxing at senior level, boxing for your country or you're about to turn professional, you could just explain to people the effects that boxing can have and just get them to think about what they want after boxing," Groves said. "It's hard to think about that when you're twenty years of age. You turn professional and you think you're going to rule the world."

Groves retired after a stoppage defeat to Callum Smith in 2019. Unlike many others, he maintained he would reject the urge to fight on but admitted, "It's hard for a boxer to let it go. It's hard to say no. It's hard to live your life if you become accustomed to being a fighter. It's not just money. It's everything that goes with it. It's hard to find any new outlet."

And Froch—who twice beat Groves before retiring—has segued into a broadcasting career after boxing. He lives well, stays healthy, and has a varied property portfolio.

"I never really thought about head injuries, I couldn't care less," Froch said. "I was always well hydrated, I was always fit and well. [Trainer] Rob McCracken always made a point of saying to keep hydrated. He'd had a career where he struggled to make weight at middleweight when he finished and he lost because he was knackered and dead at the weight. I never gave it a second thought when I was fighting. . . . And once you've been out of the sport five or ten years you see fighters who have been around, who took a lot of punishment, and I look at some of these guys and think, 'Is he a bit slow, or is he tired?' There are a few boxers who took a lot of punishment who can be associated with having a bit of a slurry voice, and they can't hold a conversation and it's a shame to see. It's very sad. But that's obviously the longer-term effect of brain injuries and impacts to the head, which I've started to think about now because I've been retired four years."

Froch continued: "I feel like my faculties are totally intact, but I like to think I keep myself busy and I keep myself active. . . . [B]ecause I'm always busy I think I will always be okay, but you never know, do you? I've been hit a couple of times where I've been shaken to my boots. I've been hit a couple of times in the head where I've been dizzy and I've been dazed, but I can only count on one hand how many times that's happened. I was put down twice in my career—Jermain Taylor and George Groves—but I got back up to win. Robin Reid hit me with a good right hand. I felt that when I went back to the corner. And a guy called Varujan Davtyan at York Hall, I walked into a right hand and when I went back to the corner I was looking at where I wanted to go but my legs were deceiving my brain and going the other way."

Froch said he couldn't recall rounds eight through ten of his twelve-round war when he first won the WBC super-middleweight title against Jean Pascal. By the time he retired, he'd boxed for twenty years, had around a hundred amateur fights, forty pro fights, and reckoned he sparred 130 rounds in preparation for most of his bigger bouts. He logged his work in detailed training diaries.

John H. Stracey, another of the finest UK boxers and the WBC's first welterweight world champion, was also doing just fine at the age of sixty-nine. While his health stood firm and he was a wonderful talker and a startlingly good singer, he noticed his contemporaries struggle badly into old age.

"There's a decline over the years," Stracey stated. "I think from the late fifties through to the seventies is where you will find the problem."

Like many boxers, he believes alcohol and drugs hasten any decline but there are other factors that led him to believe he may have dodged the neurological bullet. "I retired at twenty-eight, I'd had fifty-one pro fights and I'd won thirty-seven out of forty-five inside the distance. So if you take all the rounds I should have done—say I should have done 510 rounds over fifty-one fights—I'd done 284, so there were well over 200 rounds that I didn't do. If I had done them, we don't know how I would have been. [And] we never sparred hard. I give my manager Terry Lawless his due there. He would say, 'Hey, don't start killing each other in training, you do that when you fight.' So we sort of three-quarter fought, which is the best, because you're not going full out."

For Stracey, early education was key, but he still thought the macho culture of the sport meant any lessons learned might be forgotten when toughness is summoned. "When you go to a gym where there are a lot of good fighters, they all want to show off that they're the best so they're going to try and kill you, but you need someone saying, 'Hey lads, you're not getting paid for this at the moment, wait until your fight. Then you do it.'"

Stracey regularly attended functions with older fighters. He is in Canastota at the International Boxing Hall of Fame each year, he moves up and down the United Kingdom as an after-dinner speaker, often along-side boxers of his vintage. "What happens is some you see who have declined, they probably think they're okay but you can sense a decay in them," he sighed. "I'm in great [condition] but we don't know in ten years how I will be. No one can prophesize that, but now I'm still able to do things and run and train if I want. I think we all know that there could be issues. I wasn't silly enough to think something may not happen."

And Stracey, who won his world title in sensational fashion, knocking out Mexican idol Jose Napoles in a bullring in Mexico in 1968, has seen plenty of once-proud and ambitious fighters lose their way, their focus, and, ultimately, their minds. "It's never been properly addressed," he added. "It's shocking. I've seen a few fighters over the years who are really bad, some don't even remember me and I've been great friends with them. We've got to educate, that's what we need to do, and when they retire we've got to help people. But what happens is when someone retires they say, 'Oh good, now I will do what I like.' And then they go into more problems [with alcohol, drugs, and living excessively]. Years ago we didn't know. Now we know what the problems are [and] we can deal with them, and that's the great thing about it."

One of the all-time great punchers, Julian Jackson, who chomped on a few sticks of dynamite himself while dishing out his own TNT, winning fifty-five of sixty-one fights and losing all six by knockout, believed that, at nearly sixty years of age, he was in good shape because he was dedicated and lived a well-disciplined life.

"I have my health because I respected the sport and the sport respected me," he said, talking about shying away from a party lifestyle and drink and drugs. "If you treat the sport right, then it will treat you right."

Lennox Lewis, the great heavyweight king, walked away a millionaire and lives a happy life in retirement. He waited until the end of his boxing journey to get married and have children, he didn't want to have a civilian life while being a prizefighter so he put boxing first.

In trainer Emanuel Steward, he had a wise head to educate him about both the intricacies and the risks of the sport. "We used to call it 'walking on your heels,'" Lewis said, as he recalled another term that was used to describe CTE. "They need to address it in all sports, even in soccer. It should be addressed because obviously it can lead to suicide down the line and a number of other illnesses, like Parkinson's."

The potential for long-term health problems for him is not something he ever considers. "No," he confessed. "There's nothing I think about like that because boxing, when I first started, people were saying, 'What about Muhammad Ali?' That's what made me say, 'I have to retire at a certain time and I have to make sure that I don't get hit.' I wanted to be a thrower, not a catcher. Those things were always in my mind when I was boxing. It's interesting, there's two types of fighters. There's catchers and there's pitchers. The catchers are the ones that will go through that because they're taking punishment all the time and getting knocked out and it's sad, but if you step in the ring there can only be one champion, and you've just got to make sure that you're the one champion. You've got to make sure that you don't take the punches. You've got to make sure that you look after your life. People around you that you trust, such as your cornermen and your family, need to be part of that life so they can say, 'Hey, listen, I think you're taking too much. I don't think you should take any more fights.' That's how serious the sport is. My mum was fully involved with my boxing in the sense that she knew if I was taking shots."

And while Lewis said Steward would not condone his having wars, Steward instilled a toughness into Lewis through sparring, hard sparring at that. He credited that type of training with his getting through ten tough rounds with fellow 1988 Olympic gold medalist Ray Mercer in New York's Madison Square Garden.

"That's why I won that fight," Lewis admitted. "I boxed three tough guys, Philly fighters, tough guys, and they just rushed me. Manny [Steward] would give us a minute and we would go hard, hard, hard. Then stop. Then he'd throw another guy in and you'd have to adjust and go hard, hard, hard. These guys don't get tired, they were pushing me to get tired."

It is that hard and fast combat environment that those hurt by the sport contend needs to change, but it's the one thing New York's former welterweight world champion Paulie Malignaggi, who has become a notable broadcaster in retirement, would never sacrifice. "Yeah, that's not going to happen," he said, of toning down sparring. "If you're going to prepare yourself for a fight, you're going to have to spar a lot of rounds; otherwise you're not going to be sharp. Doctors have to be doctors but fighters have to be fighters also. That's also the problem—it's hard to intermingle the two."

Then there is the fact that fighters are taught to be tough. Rarely when asked whether they are okay to continue in a fight, be it by a trainer or referee, will the fighter say no. On the contrary, some instruct their corner to never throw in the towel, and then say they would rather die in the ring than face the "shame" of defeat or being withdrawn.

"You have to mask the injuries and the pain," Malignaggi went on. "You always consider brain trauma and whatnot, but I was not super educated in it and you don't worry about it until it happens. If you start thinking about it, you'll be thinking about it all the time. Especially when I was fighting, I didn't think about this kind of thing. I've had fights where I don't remember the end of them. You're definitely going to get a concussion. If you're going to box, you're going to wind up with concussion. If you're going to be in contact sports, you're going to wind up with concussion. You're going to take damage, so you try to avoid as much damage as you can. I was defensive because I was good enough to be defensive. I think fighters that could be defensive would probably choose to be. I don't think everybody chooses to be aggressive all the time unless they have no other choice."

Malignaggi has heard all the terms the sport's critics use, from primitive to barbaric. He thinks they just don't understand boxing and he pays no attention to it. The attention given to trauma in other sports, however, has caused Malignaggi to think about his contemporaries, particularly those suffering from depression, personality changes, and mood swings.

"They see the boxers and they think it's from winding up with no money or whatever," he said. "I think some of it starts with the brain trauma you receive. Look at Jermain Taylor. I was signed to the same stable as Jermain Taylor for years and he was a totally normal guy. After his retirement, he was shooting guns up in the air and all that kind of stuff so, you know, I think the brain trauma can be linked to some of these fighters, it's just nobody does their research."

Mexican legend Marco Antonio Barrera said that he had done his. Barrera had a craniotomy in 1997, a procedure that was completed after his second bout with Junior Jones, though not because of it. The surgery was done to remove an unusual vein, so doctors opened up his skull, took out the vein, and placed metal plates around it, fixing it with screws inside his skull. He went on to fight his best, wildest fights after the surgery in his long, decorated Hall of Fame career.

"I have had two plates in my head for twenty-two years since the surgeries," he said in 2018. "It's dangerous but if you have a good doctor and you check regularly, it's not dangerous. I fought all my big fights after the surgeries. I fought Erik Morales three times, Naseem Hamed, [Juan Manuel] Marquez, and my head is fine and I feel very good."

Whether or not Barrera was rolling the dice more than other fighters, we don't know. He was subsequently licensed to fight in Texas, California, Nevada, England, and China before finishing his incredible seventy-five-fight career.

Youngstown middleweight champion Kelly Pavlik boxed forty-two times as a professional and retired on the back of four wins. "When I quit, I promised my kids at a young age and my wife that I was going to be done," he said. "They wanted me to be done shortly after I won the world title and that [CTE]'s a big thing. Even to this day, I still worry about it. I don't know what's going to happen.

He continued: "What people don't understand is, it's not the fights. Fights are the glamorous part that people see. Where the damage comes in, especially in the old days when they really didn't understand, it comes in three, four days a week sparring. Some of these guys are doing like three hundred rounds in camp. I can't remember what I did, but it was minimum a hundred rounds in camp and sparring was full go. I mean, I've seen more people get knocked out, dropped, stopped in sparring, and that's where the damage comes."

From his amateur days, Pavlik would sometimes spar as much as four days a week and he piled up the rounds in eight-week training camps as a professional.

"Should they stop it [boxing]? No," he said. "Fighters know what they're getting into and it's the same thing with football, they know what they're signing up for when they go into it. But I think there should be some more research into it. It's scary. It truly is. I have a guy close to me and I could see the shaking, the trembles in his hand.

"It's hard even if you do the research. If you put headgear on, it's still trauma. If you do the tests after the fight, the damage is already done. What do you really do for something like that? After a twelve-round fight? What makes boxing more dangerous than MMA, say, as happened with me against [Jermain] Taylor, you get dropped in the second round, you've got ten seconds. In MMA they stop the fight, which they should, the guy could get killed. But in boxing if you get up and you're good, you're in a competitive fight and say you get dropped again and you get a referee who's lenient and you get up under the ten-second count you can get dropped three or four times in a fight. Your brain's scrambled already and you can still go twelve rounds or thirty-six minutes with a brain injury. What is research going to show you after a fight like that? What is research going to do if in sparring when you're bringing in former world champions and professional sparring partners and you're sparring ten, twelve rounds? So on the research—unless they find cures for it, or a blockage of killing of brain cells or what causes dementia—how are you going to stop it?"

British boxing pundit and broadcaster Steve Bunce has seen fighters change over time and their outlooks become more grim. He has a slightly different theory about how much a fighter can put into the sport—how much punishment they can take and over how long. He sees that there are limits.

"Inside your body, you have a box, and in that box you have your boxing life, and that box gets depleted like a gas tank," he theorized. ". . . and that keeps going down and down and down until you're running on empty. And fighters that run on empty are not necessarily guys like Peter Buckley who had three hundred fights or guys like [135-fight American veteran] Bruce 'The Mouse' Straus. Sometimes a guy can be running on empty if he's had nineteen, twenty-nine, or thirty fights. Think about Vernon Sollis. I think he was twenty-two when his career was over and he was knocked out cold by someone in the Midlands, but he should not have been in that state. He was 'gone' then, at twenty-two years of age having won the British title. It's not black-and-white."

Bunce is an old-school boxing stalwart. His face creased awkwardly when the words "punch-drunk" were mentioned. It is not a topic anyone relishes discussing. "I think I used the word 'gone' to describe a punch-drunk fighter for the first time," he claimed. "I was talking about Herol Graham when he fought Vinny Paz. He'd passed all the tests. He'd actually been out to California to pass some cognitive tests, not just to see if his brain was clear, and, unfortunately, he's just 'gone.' But it [being 'gone'] isn't talked about it and if you do talk about it, people get a bit upset with you for mentioning it, for suggesting it. I work with a lot of fighters on TV and radio who I would classify as a little bit 'gone,' and, let's be brutally honest, I've heard their slurs increase during the tail end of their careers. Over the last twenty-five years, I've heard hundreds of boxers' voices deteriorate and seen their mental abilities drop a level or two. Strangely, I've also seen dozens of boxers improve when they stop fighting, their voices become clearer over a period of time, so it is something that's swept under the table because it's not something that's instant. It doesn't happen overnight."

Bunce had about sixty fights out of the Fitzroy Lodge Amateur Boxing Club in London. He was stopped once, dropped only a couple of times, and doesn't consider now whether his health may falter due to the shots he took.

And officials in boxing should be mindful too, he continued. Bunce often calls for fights to be stopped before the officials get around to doing it because he is aware of the long-term dangers that lurk. He has seen the toll boxing has taken on fighters, especially at gatherings of retired boxers a few years removed from the prize ring.

"There's things like the London Ex-Boxers," he said. "It's brilliant to see all those guys, but ten years ago X was okay and now X is in real trouble and he's still only seventy. When you go back to those gatherings some of the guys reached a decent level, some of them were anonymous [never made it to the top], so technically are they punchy? I don't know. But I would consider them 'gone,' yes. If they were still boxing and they were thinking about boxing, would I tell the [British Boxing] Board [of Control]? Yes. And in my life I've probably mentioned to the Board about thirty boxers who I thought shouldn't fight. We're in the gyms when we're not being paid and you're there to speak to one fighter and you end up speaking to ten others and it's during those sessions where you encounter those fighters and you think, 'Fucking hell, he shouldn't be fighting anymore.' And it's not necessarily guys who have lost twenty-eight out of thirty-two. There's no direct correlation."

But his concerns aren't just at the top end of the scale. He worries about amateurs too, as well as changes in the system that mean some fighters are emerging from the amateur ranks with as many as three hundred fights behind them. International teams have full-time training camps and high-quality sparring, and bouts in some events are now five three-minute rounds rather than the more traditional three two or three-minute rounds. The headgear has also gone. There has been talk of decorated amateurs turning professional and already showing signs of taking too much punishment.

"You ain't joking," said Bunce. "World Series of Boxing. APB [AIBA Pro Boxing]. Full-on training camps. Full-on sparring. Two years of it. Seventy or eighty fights. Twenty-odd fights a year over five rounds. There's a lot of fighters at the moment that are cruising through the early pro years that have done all their work already, and I fear for them. That's a real problem," he said.

One fighter who boxed plenty before turning pro was Team Great Britain star Tony Jeffries, who captured a bronze in the 2008 Olympics but then had his professional career curtailed by hand injuries. It is something he is happy about now. He has a successful gym in California, teaching celebrities, kids, MMA athletes, and professional and amateur boxers how to fight. But CTE is a hot topic for him and he has his own fears. He is part of the fighter study in Las Vegas and has worked out that he's been punched approximately fifty thousand times in the head. He totaled 106 fights in his career, pro and amateur, and used that sum to work backward.

"Let's say I averaged four rounds a fight, that's 424 rounds I've fought," Jeffries started. "Now, let's say for each of those rounds I was hit in the head seven times—I know it was more sometimes and fewer others—that's 2,968 times I've been punched from my fights. So, if I sparred ten times for each fight, and each spar was six rounds, that would mean I'd sparred 6,360 rounds. Now, stay with me here, seven headshots in each round would mean I'd received 44,520 blows to the head. I started boxing when I was ten, but before I fought I had to spar—and spar a lot back then. I used to only spar around four rounds at a time and this was three times a week. It was about four months of boxing training before I had my first fight aged eleven. Four rounds, three times a week comes to twelve rounds a week. If you multiply that by five months, it works out at 240 rounds sparring. Now, at this age when I was learning, let's say I was hit ten times each round, it meant I was punched in the head around 2,400 times aged just eleven."

You get the picture Jeffries is painting. How many times does an ordinary person recall being banged on the head? Maybe once when they stood up quickly somewhere there was a low ceiling, or when they fell off their bike while learning to ride, or perhaps even in a drunken punch-up. But fighters take blows to the head repeatedly, often several days a week. That, for many, is where the real danger lies.

So thirty-five-year-old Jeffries waits. He panics when he forgets something. If he gets angry, he wonders if it's CTE beginning to bite, or if he gets down whether it's tightening its grip. It's the unknown.

And worry he does. "Big time," he said. "I think about it all the time. Like now, if I misplace my car keys or can't find anything I think, 'Shit, is this a sign of dementia?' If I stumble over some words I'm saying, which I do sometimes, I put it down to boxing."

Maybe it has taken the NFL's concussion crisis for a few people in boxing to take note, or maybe once you've been in the sport a certain amount of time, you realize what it can do and what it can take from its protagonists.

Nigel Collins is the former editor of *The Ring*, covered the sport for more than forty years, and was inducted into the International Boxing Hall of Fame. He has seen it all, including the first fight between light-heavyweight greats Matthew Saad Muhammad and Marvin Johnson in 1977 which was so violent that he thought, from ringside, that both boxers might die that night.

"My feelings about boxers getting brain damage has changed a lot over the years," he admitted. "I now believe that a minimum 75 to 80 percent suffer some kind of brain damage. Some of it is very severe, some of it is not that bad. But it could be more than 80 percent—I'm not sure—but it's rare that they get out in one piece."

Yet for all of the tragedy and heartbreak, Collins said he had never met a fighter who said they wouldn't do it all again. Boxing becomes their identity and the toll will continue to rise.

"I'm used to what the fighters look like," Collins said, "but I went up to Canastota [to the International Boxing Hall of Fame] one year with somebody who'd never been before but was a boxing fan and he was mortified when he saw all of these broken-down people, and that some of them could hardly speak. That was a real shock to him. People have asked me about becoming boxers and I say, 'You're going to get brain damage. It's cut and dried.'"

17
Safety Nets

HELP AFTER THE FINAL BELL

There's a seventy-three-year-old with big dreams and grand ambitions.

David Harris has followed boxing since the 1970s and he is spearheading Ringside Rest and Care, an initiative that could benefit dozens of old boxers in the United Kingdom. The plan is to build a care home where ex-professionals can be looked after, where they can retell stories of their careers and be surrounded by colleagues in the same situation.

"This is going to be a world leader because I tell you what, I won't rest until it's done," pledged Harris. Indeed, the fundraising efforts have seen people of all ages travel far and wide. "We've had people climb Mt. Blanc, someone's climbing Kilimanjaro, we've done parachute jumps, little clubs like Northolt [Amateur Boxing Club] gave a thousand pounds, a club of seven- to ten-year-olds raised £300 in a walk, there's something happening every week," he went on. "We struggled in the first few months, but I wrote 1,179 letters to every amateur club in the country asking for their support. The professionals have not been nearly as great but there are pockets of real support, like Wales, in the Valleys, the support from there has been astronomical but it's tough. We've tried major promoters and I asked for a pound to be added to each ticket sold that could go to the Ringside Rest and Care Home. That fell on deaf ears."

Ringside Rest and Care was awarded charity status in late 2019, meaning it came closer to being realized. Harris has been told that by the time the charity had two years of audited accounts, then bigwig investors from London will intervene and help the project not only over the line but assist as it moves forward.

While Harris won't take credit for the idea, given that rest homes for fighters have been talked about for decades, he is the driving force behind it. "I don't know if it's my brainchild because when I first came into professional boxing they were saying then 'We've got to do something' and nobody ever did. And I know why—because it takes a lot of hard work. Our plan is to have a place that's going to have a cinema room, it's going to have hairdressers, a non-alcoholic bar where they can sit and talk in the evenings if they want to, and the carers will know all their records and they'll be able to pull up their fight films so they can see their old contests."

Like so many in the sport, Harris is keen to maintain the respect the fighters have earned. That means being sympathetic to their plights without using old-school vernacular, such as "punch-drunk syndrome."

"We cover every aspect of damage to boxers because there's alcohol-related diseases, there's brain damage of different types, and there's a lot of dementia that seems to be coming earlier in boxers' lives, so when they're forty or fifty a lot of them are starting to suffer," he explained. "Dementia pugilistica is what they keep hitting me with. What I'm trying to do is say, 'Yes, we've got a problem.' We know the risks in boxing, what we want to do is be there for those who fall through the net, and that's the nicest way of saying it."

Harris knew of thirty-eight old fighters who needed residential care, the majority of them required it round the clock. His team includes a treasurer, legal experts, business aides and trustees, raising funds and keeping his improbable dream alive until the financial cavalry arrives. "They're coming on board big style," he said optimistically of the stock-market investors and monied people who have promised their substantial involvement.

While there's merit to what Harris is trying to do, the crisis runs far deeper than thirty-eight lost souls. It's at the core of the sport and it's a global issue. Mauricio Sulaiman, head of the World Boxing Council (WBC), is aware of CTE and the long-term health implications of the sport. He often hosts award dinners with dozens of champions present, and he attends big fights and functions where he sees the toll the sport has taken. But the wider problem is neither his nor the WBC's. The WBC looks out for its champions and those who have boxed for their belts. Sulaiman also helps some older fighters who have never won WBC titles with handouts, but he cannot see boxing uniting to confront CTE.

"I feel terrible because it's very sad to see a great hero from the past in difficulty," Sulaiman said, citing that football players, rock stars, and actors and actresses also struggle when they are no longer at the top. "Every star in a sport or in entertainment goes through a very difficult and challenging time when success, fame, money, and glory comes. That's the private life. A boxer who has a decent, healthy life outside the ring will most likely not suffer consequences as we have seen happening. We are working very hard on the awareness side with young boxers. We are trying to limit sparring rounds. We are recommending many things to try and keep a good life. There is a stigma but people who do need help don't want to talk about it. When you have CTE you are sick, and there are certain treatments that can help in certain ways. We are addressing it, we aren't hiding from it, on the contrary."

And to their credit, the WBC has a history of exploring and implementing safety measures. It works with Dr. Charles Bernick at the Cleveland Clinic, it has sent fighters to join his fighter study, and Mauricio's late father, Jose Sulaiman—who was in power before Mauricio—looked at improving fighter safety back in the 1970s.

"The WBC recognized the issue a long time ago," Mauricio continued. "My father came from a small town in Mexico—his friends were boxers, that's how he got involved—and he went through the whole ladder from being an amateur boxer to ring announcer to trainer, referee, judge, assistant, supervisor, everything in boxing he did at one time of his life. And when he was in the position to make changes in the sport, he immediately did that. . . . [M]y father met with UCLA, the hospital, which has great prestige, and the WBC funded a study in 1978. Eventually, in a two-year period, the government of the United States provided $50 million to UCLA to continue with what they had found. With that research in boxing came the change from fifteen to twelve rounds, the change of the day of the weigh-in from one day before, the weight management of the sport. The six-ounce gloves were banned, medical examinations were made mandatory, which before did not exist, there were suspensions after knockouts. So if we do an analysis of the rules in 1970 and how throughout the years they were modified, that is the response. We do recognize it. We believe the mental health of the current fighters is much better than the older fighters because of these changes."

It's easy to blame the splintered nature of the sport because boxing needs federal reform. Senator John McCain was an advocate of a national boxing commission in the United States to at least have each state singing off the same hymn sheet, but even that would be just one country in a world where few seem to willingly operate in synchronicity.

"Unfortunately there's an issue that interferes with that, which is law," Sulaiman continued. "And each country has their own laws—the UK, the United States, Mexico, Russia, Japan. . . . In the United States, each state has a different law. And when you discuss topics of medicine, medicals, the law prohibits the information to be public, in a way, so that is one of the major obstacles that we face. If we go to a jurisdiction which has a different policy then it's up to each jurisdiction [to enforce regulations], but for the WBC, all we can do is recognize a fight."

They can also only intervene with WBC sanctioned fights, even though their research does benefit others in the sport.

However, of all the fights that take place around the world each week, the WBC, WBA, IBF, and WBO are involved in only a fraction. They have nothing to do with club shows or small events unless one of their titles is on the line, so why would they help a fallen fighter they've never done business with or who has never paid a sanctioning fee?

The WBC, however, like the NFL, is seen as one of the sport's power brokers. Is Sulaiman worried about fighters suing the sanctioning body down the line, the same way players gunned for the NFL? In a word, no. "It's very different because the NFL, as a league, is the owner of everything that happens," he said. "They own the TV rights, they own the teams, they sell the franchises, they own everything that has to do with their sport, so there's a natural conflict of interest. In each of the other sports—baseball, soccer, football, hockey, basketball—those leagues are the ones that make the business and make the rules so there's an internal conflict. In boxing it's different, the sport is controlled by the promoters. They are the ones that make the business, they contract the fighters, they contract the venues, they contract the sponsors, the television networks, and then the organization just comes in to sanction and regulate one specific fight, not each of the fights. So it's different."

Different states, different bodies, different countries. No wonder fighters fall through the cracks. At the British Boxing Board of Control, there is a grant that helps boxers who have started to struggle. It's an annual pool, made up from fundraising and fines through the years that is distributed around Christmas to fighters in need. A few hundred pounds here, a few hundred there. It's nothing that alleviates symptoms or helps pave the way forward for a new beginning, but it's a gesture nonetheless.

Robert Smith is a former fighter and the general secretary of the British Boxing Board of Control. Since taking the top job in 2009, he's introduced new measures to increase safety, including a two-day trainer's course that has a first-aid module. Scanning protocols have also changed.

"I think a lot of people probably don't want to admit that they have an issue themselves," he said of older fighters. "I think people in the sport previously have brushed it under the carpet for whatever reason but it's something we are well aware of. I hate the term *punch-drunk*—it's CTE now and it is a concern. I boxed. Would I be the same person if I hadn't boxed? I don't know. My father had seven amateur fights and at the end of his life suffered with Alzheimer's and dementia. Did boxing do that to him? I don't know. My granddad had two hundred fights and he suffered from dementia. Did boxing do that to him? You'd guess it didn't help. My auntie, my dad's sister, never had a fight in her life and she suffered from dementia, so it's very difficult to pinpoint it as just boxing. But I am realistic that taking punches to the head ultimately doesn't do you any good. I don't know what more we can do with the measures we've put in place and the meetings I'm having and the people I'm talking to [in order to] try and tweak the rules, regulations, and medical standards."

Smith is an old-fashioned man. He worked as an engineer through his fighting days, running in the early morning, going to work by day, and training at the boxing gym in the evening. He was 14-1 when he took a late-notice call to fight future world champion Lloyd Honeyghan at London's Royal Albert Hall. But he had a trade to fall back on, and with the Honeyghan payout he put himself on a business-studies course to pave the way for his future. He had foresight many fighters don't have or use, and that's why he's a little short on sympathy when a boxer doesn't have a plan B. He sees them as self-employed, and that when one job finishes they should know that they will have to take on another.

Of course, it's not as simple as all that, particularly if they have put their lives on hold to focus on the sport or if they're damaged as a consequence of chasing that dream.

A lot of Smith's job is red tape, legal wrangles about licensing fighters, performance-enhancing-drug cases, and disciplinary action. He'd rather be governing the sport than knee-deep in court cases each day, but that's what the role has become. And he does worry about CTE case after CTE case knocking on his door, hand open, or legal letters posting claim after claim against the Board.

"Hand on heart, yes," he admitted. "I think society has changed. We do have a blame culture; people have to take their own responsibilities. Nobody is dragged into a boxing ring and made to fight. They get in there of their own free will, as I did, but as a responsible organization we have to make it as safe as we possibly can, and I think we have."

The lack of support for fighters has been felt over the years, and it has inspired boxers to help their own. Former great lightweight champ Beau Jack, who wound up shining shoes in Miami, attempted to get a pension plan in place but by then he was a forgotten man. In the United Kingdom, former world featherweight champion Barry McGuigan tried to start a union, the Professional Boxers' Association, with fellow ex-boxers Nicky Piper, a Commonwealth light-heavyweight champion, and former WBO featherweight ruler Colin McMillian. That was in 1993. The goal was to provide fighters with a bridge of support as they crossed into life after boxing, whether it was with counseling or advice. McGuigan tried in vain for fifteen years to make it work.

There are plenty in boxing who would say that active pros wouldn't listen to advice anyway. Life for them is for the now, the next fight. Too many boxers think they will get in, make a fortune, and get out. Smith recommended a pension plan for boxers in the United Kingdom for a while. Not one active pro paid into it.

Former heavyweight contender Gerry Cooney, a great white hope in the 1980s, set up a foundation to support retired fighters, but FIST (Fighters' Initiative for Support and Training) was plagued with issues. Still, he recognized then as he does now that ex-boxers need help. "Now the part that bothers me is the teachers [trainers]," he said, of how the sport should adapt. "There shouldn't be guys with twelve-ounce gloves slugging it out in the gym in training, they should wear twenty-four-ounce gloves. When the tires wear out on your car, you change them, but in your body you can't, so you've got to be very careful."

Cooney argued that the problem with boxing is the managers and the promoters. "They don't want to educate the fighters on how to take care of themselves so they pay their laundry, they pay their rent, they pay their insurance because they want to feel, 'Hey, I got this guy. This guy's with me.' But the problem is when he becomes twenty-eight or thirty and the world championships are not there anymore, now you become a sparring partner and an opponent, they move on to somebody else and the fighter's left alone. I tell everyone, 'Go to the commission where you live and learn what you're signing. Understand it. Learn. Teach yourself.' We have to protect ourselves and you've got to be careful because when you're young you don't pay attention to it. . . . It's a sad story because you see the fans cheering but the fighters are killing themselves. They're beating themselves to death."

It is the transition into a new life where FIST really tried to help, but Cooney found difficulties. Fighters who had headlined big TV shows and who had achieved a level of fame weren't so enamored by the prospect of a nine-to-five. "We had a lot of good success with FIST, but the problem was the guys didn't really want to work, they wanted money," Cooney said. "Now you figure they get out of high school, they're fighting, they're not catching up with life. So now they're thirty to thirty-two and they don't know how to do it and they're too lazy to do it and there are other problems. There's drug and alcohol dependency, there's family, there's wives, legal problems, and there's so many things you can list. We did a great job for a long time but it was very difficult. Ninety-nine percent of fighters end up broke and depressed and not happy, and it's because at the end of the day they feel lost, nobody helps them fill up on the inside. There's no happiness in the fight game. I had a great career. Did I get to where I wanted to go? No, but I enjoyed every minute of what I did. I had so many great moments in my life. So did those guys but they don't appreciate it anymore because they feel like boxing turned its back on them, and in a lot of ways it does."

While FIST came and went, so did JAB [Joint Association of Boxers] headed by former light-heavyweight champion Eddie Mustafa Muhammad, despite their linkup with the Teamsters. Alex Ramos, a middleweight from the 1980s, wound up living on the streets, cleaning up in rehab before setting up the Retired Boxers Foundation, which has helped many fighters. Boxers often need help, but no one has made that huge breakthrough to help the sport on a large scale.

Matt Farrago is another ex-fighter trying to help. "The Beta Bomber," from the Bronx, won twenty-five bouts as a pro, lost just two, and drew one. In 2011 he helped form the nonprofit organization Ring 10. Farrago's mission statement is this: "Unlike other major sports that have a union to represent the athlete, professional boxers have no such safety net. Even without a union it is hard to believe that legendary fighters such as Mickey Walker, Sandy Saddler, Kid Gavilan, Ken Norton, and Joe Frazier would not be taken care of by the organized-boxing establishment when they fell on hard times after retiring from the ring. But, unfortunately, that is the case. We are proud to say that Ring 10 of New York is stepping up and making a difference with assistance and contributions to all impoverished and/or ailing fighters [regardless of background or origin]."

CTE is a subject close to Farrago's heart. He is suffering too, and he also endures the stigma from the *punch-drunk* terminology. Even though the label has changed, the stereotype remains.

"I totally agree because fighters don't suffer from CTE, they're just 'punchy,'" he said, cynically. "What the hell does that mean? We don't suffer from CTE, we're 'punchy'? But that's okay? Give them a lollipop and put them in the corner and he'll be okay because he's 'punchy'? You see, they've gotten away with it for a hundred years. We knew about dementia pugilistica—that's the proper way to say it, not pugilistic dementia, boxer's dementia—we've known about it for a hundred years and we've never been taken seriously until football came out with CTE. Oh, unbelievable, a medical term. *Chronic traumatic encephalopathy*. But we don't suffer from that because we're different. When we get punched in the head, it's not the same as two helmets hitting each other, right? Really? Bullshit, because it's camouflaged and boxing doesn't want to acknowledge it because we only become 'punchy,' it's not so bad. It's even kind of cute. I'm being sarcastic."

Farrago is desperate to educate people about the dangers. He's involved in clinical trials in New York, Las Vegas, Boston, and Florida and he's trying to get other fighters involved in the studies, too, if for nothing else than to make sure they're aware about what is happening to them. He's dealing with CTE and it's changed his life. He's fifty-eight and fears for his future. Through Ring 10 he has helped homeless fighters get back on their feet, but he's seen plenty of them deteriorate, too.

"They're all going to be rich," Farrago shrugged, going back over the start of a fighter's journey. "Everybody's going to be a world champion. Everybody's going to retire a champion and be wealthy. Well, first of all, even if you did become a champion, probably 95 percent of champions go broke within a year or two. Same with football. I don't know the exact statistic but within about three years, they're broke. But [do you know what] the big difference between a professional basketball player, a professional football player, a professional hockey player, a professional baseball player, and a fighter is? The most profound difference? Where do all of them come from before they turn pro? They come from college and [they have] college scholarships. Where does a fighter come from? They come from the streets. Now he's champion of the world—he's got money, he's got fame, and everything else. As soon as he loses, he's going back to the streets. If he didn't save anything, he's got nothing and nobody wants him. One of my board of directors is Iran Barkley, who is a five-time world champion, defeated Tommy Hearns, fought Duran, fought them all. We found him homeless on the street. Literally homeless."

Farrago doesn't like to name the names of the fighters he has helped, but it's known that Ring 10 makes regular payments to long-term boxing victims Wilfred Benitez and Gerald McClellan. They've been trying to support both of them for the nine years they've been in existence.

But the illness is still disregarded. CTE remains a diagnosis under one's breath, muttered in the shadows or on the periphery of social events. "Most fighters won't even acknowledge it," Farrago added. "If you really had the time, the money, and the effort, you could calculate how many fighters are divorced because most women will not put up with the symptoms and what the fighters are going through. My wife was an angel and she put up with it for as long as she did and then couldn't take it anymore and she was gold. She just couldn't take it anymore. So that's one of the side effects of CTE. . . . You forget, you have mood swings, you're irritable, it's not a good thing to have and you have it for life. And boxing won't take credit for it because we're only 'punchy.' Who am I going to give credit [to], or who's going to take responsibility [for] this? The NFL was easy. Finally they got a lawsuit and they acknowledged that, 'Yes, we knew of the head trauma many years ago, we withheld that information.' But it was the NFL, the National Football League. Who's going to do that in boxing? Who's going to be sued? Don King?"

And then we come again to the lack of an umbrella organization, governing the sport from top to bottom, making it safer across the board and helping those up after they have fallen. For Farrago, that's a pipe dream, even if it is one he has previously chased.

"No one in boxing is going to fund that kind of change," he said. "Everybody's got a piece of the fighters, but nobody is taking responsibility for them. There is no national or international commission, so anybody can do what they want, it's a free-for-all, it's the Wild West of sports, the last of the sports to be treated like this. It has to be done because the sport is brutal: they use them, abuse them, and then lose them. That's my signature quote for what the sport does for their fighters."

Over the years, many individuals have tried to help the masses. The McGuigans, Cooneys, Farragos, and others all saw enough but were powerless to stop boxing's broken from crashing upon wave after wave of tragedy. Thousands have slipped through the cracks with no safety net, as Farrago said, used, abused, and lost.

18
Tequila for Breakfast

SPARRING, QUITTING, RETIREMENT, DEPRESSION

eal fighters don't quit.

In fact, that's the dirtiest word in the sport. If you're losing, go out on your shield. If you're afraid, don't show it. If you're hurt, disguise it. If you can't win, deal with it.

But don't quit. Not ever.

That's unless you're damaged goods, over the hill, "shot," or "gone." Then quit, quit the sport and don't let the door hit you on the way out. The problem is by the time that part comes, the time to walk away, fighters don't know how to quit. They can't give up. Their financial future might not be secure. They might not have that title yet. They might not have anything to go to. They might know nothing else. They can't just quit, even though by the time they start actually thinking about it, it's probably already too late.

Even the chosen few who do go out on their own terms struggle. They miss the limelight, the buzz, the identity. It's like the Superman movie where Clark Kent gives up his powers. He becomes mortal. He's the same as everyone else. He's no longer the fighter, the guy on TV, the hardest guy in the room. He's just a man. He's not the one that thousands watch, just one that thousands ignore. "He is" becomes "he used to be" or "he was." A somebody becomes a nobody, maybe not to everyone but to himself, and that's more damaging and hurtful.

Joe Calzaghe never lost a professional fight. He retired how he wanted and when he wanted. He was 46-0, a two-weight world champion and a future International Boxing Hall of Famer. The Welshman was one of Britain's finest fighters. Yet he hated having to turn his back, even though he knew it was the right thing to do.

"You miss the euphoria, the buzz, the adrenaline, that was my escapism," he said. "That was my self-worth, that's who I was, to me. I was a fighter and that's what I was really good at. It was my safest place. I was bullied at school."

Calzaghe fell victim to a couple of media stings, tried drugs, and came off the rails for a while. He stabilized but remembered the hard days with rawness and candor. "It's tough," he went on. "It's really tough. [I'd been] boxing since the age of eight, retired on my own terms, retired undefeated. How many boxers can say that? I beat all the top fighters I could beat at the time, won all the belts I wanted to win, and it's tough, because when you give that up it's not that easy to find something else you love."

Calzaghe has opened up to counselors over the years and said the worst thing anyone can do is act as if it doesn't exist. But that's what fighters are taught. He knows that. "Oh you can't be depressed, you're not allowed to be sad," he said, adding, "We are all human. That's the problem. We've all been through it."

The Welshman doesn't claim to know the answers and said that depression affects athletes from all sports. "It's hard to speak to somebody about what we do when you've had the biggest high that you can have and having that identity and going to these arenas and then retiring at a young age," Calzaghe said. "At the end of the day you need to move on, be proactive, and do something. I'm all for help, though, and I think there should be something in place for sportsmen. . . . Psychotherapists, counselors . . . I think it's needed."

Strangely only a few years after Calzaghe, an unbeaten champion at super middleweight and light heavyweight, walked away at the height of his fame, Californian Andre Ward duplicated the Welshman's unusual achievements. Also a decorated champion at 168 pounds and 175 pounds, Ward had won an Olympic gold medal in 2004 and was thirty-three when he fought his final contest. He was 32-0. Like for Calzaghe, it wasn't easy. The ring called him. There were offers to move up to cruiserweight and even heavyweight.

"It [retirement] sounds all neat and buttoned up, but it wasn't that easy," said Ward. "I didn't know how things were going to go throughout the course of my career, but, for whatever reason, even as a young kid—I'm talking ten years old—I had this thought, 'I don't want to end up like a lot of fighters end up.' They seem to go high, really high, and then all of a sudden they come crashing down. Like they start well but they don't end well. That's what drew me to Roy Jones Jr.—country boy, had swag, he'd always talk about himself in the third person and say, 'Roy Jones, I don't love the sport like that, I'm gonna get in, get out, I'm just special at it and I'm going to be fishing at my farm one day in Pensacola, Florida.' And I was like, 'Man, this dude is different. Fighters don't talk like that.' So he was the first one who gave me the thought of getting in and getting out."

Like Calzaghe, Ward was running out of mountains to scale—that was until he altered his mindset. He looked at retirement as an opponent, one he could not give into and he knew not only making the decision to retire but sticking to it would be the hardest decision of his life.

"At some point, I'm going to have to do this," he said when he came to the realization. "At some point I'm going to have to face the emotions, the pull to come back, and trying to figure out if your body can still do it and all the different things you go through, whether I'm in my prime or whether I'm forty or forty-five years old. You can't avoid it, it's just when you want to take on that task."

He had been boxing since the age of eight. His life could have taken a different path. Both parents were involved with drugs, but boxing has saved souls and has a history of wise custodians whose jobs and lives are dedicated to saving people like Ward from the street. Ward's dad took him to Virgil Hunter, a Bay Area boxing trainer. They would stay together from that day until Ward walked.

"If you love combat sports, if you love boxing, if you love fighting, if you enjoy it, I love the guy who's got to take two to give one but I also love the master," Ward, now a commentator for ESPN, stated. "And the problem in boxing is we've ostracized the master. Instead of articulating what we're seeing and letting the fans decide what they like or don't like, we try to tell the fans what they should like. 'Oh, this is boring' Well, that's the guy who's going to be speaking properly when all is said and done. Hopefully the other guy is too, but the likelihood is a lot less because he's taking two to give one. I'm thankful that when I walked into the gym for the first time, my dad was scouring for a trainer who could teach his son how to hit and not get hit. He saw Virg, who became my godfather and who's been my trainer through my whole career. He said, 'I'm a fan of Muhammad Ali, can you teach my son to hit and not get hit?' And Virg said, 'That's my specialty.' But just think if my dad was on something else. What if my dad was, 'Make my son tough, I want him to take it and dish it out?'"

Hunter always told Ward his priority was to get him home safely to his family; championships were merely a bonus. Sure, Hunter wanted to win, but not at the expense of his health.

Of course, time is a great leveler, but Calzaghe and Ward are rare ones, like Rocky Marciano (biographer Mike Stanton wrote how "The Rock" hated the idea of being punch-drunk and was upset by the ridicule fighters received because of it), but the super-middleweight and light-heavyweight double titlists are great examples of getting in, getting rich, and getting out. There are only a handful in boxing: Floyd Mayweather, Gene Tunney, Lennox Lewis, Vitali Klitschko. . . . Not many have been able to resist the lure of one last match, one last loan against their futures.

Frank Bruno won the WBC world heavyweight title at the fourth attempt, defeating Oliver McCall in Wembley Stadium. He was obligated to rematch Mike Tyson in his first defense and Tyson had beaten him six years earlier. Bruno went into the fight with eye problems, but while he ran a risk, he did so because he was being paid life-changing money. Tyson beat him again, this time in three rounds, and Bruno was in the post-boxing wilderness. It was also a place Bruno's old trainer, George Francis, had warned him about. He told Bruno that fighters suffer with depression, that boxing people in general suffer with depression. Francis later took his own life.

Bruno, having reached the summit, crashed spectacularly. He was a national hero but wound up forcibly hospitalized three times, was diagnosed as bipolar, went through an ugly divorce, was hunted by the British press (who added to his paranoia by bugging his phones), and he spent time in a living hell. Medication made him lethargic. Yet Bruno said suicide had never been an option.

At fifty-seven, he was in a better place, training each day, spending time in health clubs, and finally finding a routine and some comfort in a life without boxing. He was aware of CTE and the affects it can have on mood, too.

North Carolina neuroscientist Kevin M. Guskiewicz studied the rates of depression in NFL players. In response to a questionnaire, 269 of 2,552 athletes admitted to either a prior or present diagnosis of clinical depression. That's 11.1 percent. Those with a history of concussions and head trauma were more likely to suffer from depressive symptoms. Depression has long been associated with boxing, but not for as long as it should have been. And, like everything else in boxing, very little has been done about it, too. The awkward silence goes on.

And there are not many fighters who think CTE is the source of their depression. They blame defeats, poor management, the sport, often anyone but themselves. And all too often they have the *It won't happen to me* disposition, and before they know it, history has repeated itself. It's a lonely, isolating sport. Even peripheral figures have taken their own lives—referees, journalists, matchmakers, trainers.

Ricky Hatton was the most popular fighter in British sport who could draw 20,000 fans to watch him fight in Las Vegas but in retirement he found himself alone in his kitchen, a knife to his wrists crying through a fog of depression. All those fans were gone; he felt isolated.

We will never know if Edwin Valcro, the brutal punching Venezuelan who committed suicide after being accused of murdering his wife in 2010, was suffering from anything more than a criminal mind. His wife had been stabbed three times. He was 27-0 and a two-weight champion. Back in 2001 he'd been in a motorcycle crash that left him with a fractured skull and had needed a blood clot removed from his brain.

Middleweight legend Carlos Monzon threw his wife off a balcony while they were on holiday in Argentina and later died in a car crash while on temporary release from prison. He'd had one hundred fights by then.

We might not know how boxing altered the mind of James Butler, who's serving almost thirty years in prison. Butler was 20-5 but most known for a post-fight sucker punch of Richard Grant after losing their contest on points. Butler's gloves were removed, and as the two went to embrace, Butler knocked Grant out and broke his jaw. Butler, who was back in the ring three years later for four more fights, later murdered Sam Kellerman, brother of boxing analyst Max Kellerman. He killed him with a hammer and set fire to his apartment.

When a fighter goes off the rails these days, there might be a whisper of CTE. Jermain Taylor was a star, a 2000 Olympic bronze medalist, a country boy from Little Rock, Arkansas, well-liked, well-respected, and he became a unified middleweight champion. Then he suffered four losses in three years and was knocked out badly in three of those defeats, by Kelly Pavlik, Carl Froch, and Arthur Abraham, between 2007 and 2009.

Things changed. According to a 2009 MRI scan, he'd suffered a minor subdural hematoma, a brain bleed that can lead to a worst-case scenario. It can certainly alter moods and short-term memory. Yet after tests by the Mayo Clinic, the Nevada State Athletic Commission cleared him to fight after a two-year hiatus. Their decision—from a boxing perspective—was vindicated in 2014 when Taylor outhustled Australian veteran Sam Soliman for the IBF middleweight title.

The American never fought again, but by that point his rap sheet was almost as long as his thirty-eight-bout pro record. There were family fights. Some said he was slurring his speech. Police were called when he smashed his mother's car window. He shot a cousin—while preparing to fight Soliman—went to rehab, battered a patient (breaking his jaw), fired shots during a Martin Luther King parade, and there was more. Then he was imprisoned for failing to pay child support, violating terms of parole, and it was said he'd struggle to stand trial because of diminished "cognitive abilities."

This Taylor was unrecognizable from the popular Olympian who'd had the world at his feet, turning pro and then twice defeating the legendary Bernard Hopkins for his middleweight titles. By 2016, he faced fifty-four years in prison but instead served a six-year suspended sentence. "I'm just ready to fight," said Taylor, who had a drug and alcohol problem, as he left the court building, facing fines, court costs, the possibility of civil suits, six years of probation, drug screening, and 120 hours of community service. He was keeping the door ajar to box again. "Man, what am I supposed to do?" he said. "I have nothing else to do. I've been doing this job since I was twelve. This is my life. When I took those years off, I sat back and thought about it: What am I supposed to do?" Whether

Taylor, now forty-one, fights again or not, he's left it too late to make a sensible decision.

They say in boxing that timing is everything, and the key to a good quality of life after boxing could be the timing of when to walk away.

Three of the hardest changes to boxing's culture would be to lose the macho image (there's nothing wrong with tapping out in MMA), fighters retiring before it's too late and their health is severely impacted, and changes in sparring protocols. Not every spar has to be or should be a war—although it was for former WBO heavyweight title challenger Scott Welch.

He had twenty-six pro fights over seven years, leaving the sport at the age of thirty. He wanted to minimize the risk of any future problems. The Englishman had about thirty-five amateur fights. He fought for the WBO heavyweight title, but he did much of his work behind closed doors, sparring with top cruiserweights and heavyweights from the United Kingdom and the United States.

"I did a lot of hard sparring, what I would consider really brutal sparring," said the soft-spoken big man from Brighton. "I believed I had to try and knock someone out every day and if I didn't I wasn't very pleased with myself."

He went in with the likes of Frank Bruno, Derek Williams, Herbie Hide, and Ross Puritty among many others.

Those macho memories cause Welch to grin cheekily, but he bristles with remorse about the whole thing. "I would say that I'm damaged goods," he continued. "I'm definitely damaged from the game. I get blanks. I get mental blanks. I forget names. I'm pretty good with faces but I can't get names for love nor money."

He continued: "I used to spar with Alex Stewart. He fought [Evander] Holyfield and I became good friends with him. . . . At thirty-five he was knocked out by the Cuban [Jose Luis] Gonzalez and I told him to retire. He was slurring his speech and he was slowing down quite dramatically from the previous time sparring, and I said, 'Alex, you've got to get out of this game, mate.' And he said, 'If I can't box there is no life.' He died after he came home from work one day. He was fifty-one, fifty-two, laid on the sofa and I believe he had a brain hemorrhage and died. . . . I believe that was from boxing and the damage he sustained. He used to have wars in the gym and did so every day with Riddick Bowe in Gleason's. We weren't educated. Back then we'd have a fight on Saturday and be back in sparring on Monday.

"A lot of the American sparring partners who came over to England would put tequila on their cornflakes before they'd spar because they knew that they were going to get knocked out, they knew they were going to get damaged, so that was a way of blunting [the feeling of] what was going to happen," said Welch.

He was one of the few who admitted he was slowing, who was "getting caught with stupid shots." When his daughter was born, the stakes were too high to gamble and he stopped boxing. He was fine then but noticed changes in both his memory and speech as the years went by.

He missed the excitement—he was only thirty when he retired—but his adrenaline pumped with some bodyguard work and some acting gigs, including fighting Brad Pitt in the movie *Snatch*.

Peter Flanagan was an English journeyman welterweight in the early 1980s who retired with thirteen wins against seventeen losses and two draws and like Welch he thinks too much damage is acquired in sparring. He was diagnosed with dementia at sixty and had to hand in his driving license. Flanagan was an old-school type who saw the worst of boxing. One time he was allowed to box even though he had a bad cut by his eye that had not healed from sparring. Another time he was permitted to fight with a broken hand that was swollen so badly he could barely put the gloves on. Then he took fights he had no business even being offered and he wound up with a detached retina that went undiagnosed by all but him for years.

Flanagan now wants to raise awareness about CTE but is aware that boxing people don't like to talk about it. "They don't like to admit it, do they? I was asked to go to an amateur boxing show and do a little talk, and then they told me not to because it would be bad for the parents to see that this can happen, that you can end up with dementia," he continued.

"We had wars in sparring and we smashed holes out of each other and no one seemed to care, but all that is unnecessary when it's just sparring, throwing knockout punches and trying to hurt each other," Flanagan said.

The sport might not be able to save every fighter but it must give them the best chance of saving them from themselves. Fighters must be made to understand the cumulative toll sparring and boxing takes on them and they need to be prepared to walk away when the time comes. That is the hardest part for many fighters, and it's why the sport should do more to help as they start a new chapter.

EPILOGUE
LOST

The doorbell echoes. It is barely audible over the loud country music blaring from speakers inside. But someone heard it ring. After a delay, the music is turned down. There are loud stomps of feet on hardwood floors on the other side, and they are coming closer. Then, as they reach the other side, they stop. There is a fumbling of locks and handles for a few moments and then the door swings open. Former world heavyweight champion Leon Spinks holds it ajar with his right hand. He's wearing a trademark burgundy hat, "Leon Spinks World Heavyweight Champion 1978" is written in white over three lines.

A brief but tense period of questioning commenced.

"Leon, how are you doing?"

"Good," he replied quizzically, watching me while sloshing gum around in his open mouth. There was no smile nor a scowl. His big, open eyes looked blankly ahead, his lower jaw swung open with each chew.

"I spoke to Brenda earlier, she's expecting me."

"Right, Brenda said," he started. He took another long look at me. Then he tipped his left shoulder behind him, paving the way for me to walk by and closed the door behind us.

It was a nice home in a suburban area in Las Vegas, a good distance from the Strip that Leon used to run riot up and down. It was quiet. There was no sign of Brenda but we did have company. A black Labrador came up and checked me out.

"This motherfucker's crazy," Leon said of Sam, a lovely looking five-year-old whose sole purpose in life is to care for Leon.

I then asked about his son, Cory, a former junior-middleweight world champion, unaware of a family rift. "He alright," Leon said of Cory, pokerfaced but for the gum-chewing jaw.

"Where is he living?"

"I don't know where he at now."

"Is he still in St Louis?"

"Probably."

It was a challenge to make out what the ex-world heavyweight champion was saying. Leon's health plummeted in retirement, with displays of all the customary CTE symptoms. It culminated with a stroke in 2014 that left him fighting for his life in a coma and a recovery that spanned several agonizing months, but even then he did not return to where he was before. Like a hard fifteen-round battle, it took something out of him that won't be replaced.

Leon burst into America's consciousness as part of the incredible 1976 U.S. Olympic boxing team. Along with brother Michael, he netted gold, and within ten pro fights, he had won and lost the world heavyweight title in historic bouts with an aging if not quite decrepit Muhammad Ali. The rematch brought in a then-record $6 million at the gate alone, with Frank Sinatra and Sylvester Stallone watching from ringside and President Jimmy Carter tuning in from Camp David.

Before Leon walked to the ring as a betting underdog for the rematch, he kissed a cross and tucked it under his right sock, but his fast and hard life was beginning to catch up with him already, eight fights into his pro career.

Ali was trying to prove a point, desperately hoping to turn back a clock onlookers thought had run out on him.

Spinks had outlasted a tired Ali over fifteen rounds in their first fight, but Ali won their rematch over the same distance. The wrong had been righted after just seven months.

Then the rot set in. A few months later, Leon was bombed out in one round in Monaco by thunderous South African hitter Gerrie Coetzee. Don King then served up the 10-2-2 Leon to 37-0 Larry Holmes, who stopped him in three sessions in Detroit. Holmes, who would lose to Leon's brother Michael in two controversial fights, said he didn't want to be "walking around punched out and punch-drunk" as he considered his future.

Leon's career would never find any real momentum. He was his own worst enemy, living hard and enjoying life. He had fast cars, mink coats, and even hired Mr. T as his bodyguard. He was not big enough to match the heavyweight juggernauts, often only weighing around 200 pounds, but that's where the money was, although he wound up fighting the formidable Dwight Muhammad Qawi for the WBA cruiserweight title in 1986. It was a brutal loss in Reno, Nevada.

Leon was cruelly taunted by Qawi, a bulldozer of a former light-heavyweight champion who was on another level compared to the increasingly dilapidated Spinks, who by now was a falling star. Ex-con Qawi was ruthless. He was trying to goad Leon's brother Michael into a more lucrative fight—a rematch, given Michael had already defeated him—by publicly sacrificing poor Leon. He stuck out his tongue, gestured to him with his gloves, and helped himself to punches when he wanted. Leon bled from his mouth; Qawi smiled from his.

Referee Mills Lane eventually called off the "Camden Buzzsaw" the way a handler would summon his dog, stopping the one-sided slaughter four seconds before the end of round six. It was uncomfortable to watch. "And in another of the many crossroads fights in his career, Leon Spinks came up short," said HBO's Jim Lampley in commentary. But he paid tribute to Leon's resilience. In summarizing, he said, "There were no knockdowns in the bout. That is testimony to the heart and the courage of Leon Spinks."

That signaled a disastrous run of fights for Leon, who won just one of ten bouts from March 1986 to May 1988, boxing in Japan, Italy, and far-flung U.S. cities not associated with boxing. He was stopped or knocked out in five of those defeats. The depressing streak culminated in a thirty-three-second loss to Tony Morrison—a Canadian club fighter—on a small show in Connecticut. The woeful Morrison destruction prompted the Connecticut Athletic Commission to hit Leon with a thirty-day suspension. He would need to complete tests if he was to fight in the state again. It was May 30, 1988. Leon's then-manager said he would be informing other commissions and asking them to follow suit. But Leon slipped through the combat sport cracks. He found himself in a kickboxing-karate match in Syracuse for $15,000. John Florio and Ouisie

Shaprio, authors of *One Punch from the Promised Land*, a book on the Spinks brothers, wrote "It didn't take a martial arts expert to realize that Leon's cornermen would be doubling as pallbearers."

Ali's old fight doctor Ferdie Pacheco condemned the event, which thankfully did not happen in the end, saying. "It's almost to the point where they should be arrested for contributing to manslaughter. What do they want to do? Put Leon on a slab?"

Still, Spinks found a way to box again in 1991 after a three-year hiatus, fighting in the backwaters of Illinois, North Carolina, Washington State, and at home in St. Louis.

He was matched soft. He needed to be, and he won his first five against opponents with combined records of 52-92-5 but he was soon back in the "L" column when outscored by 13-8-2 Kevin P. Porter. Leon didn't take the hint and besides, he had nothing else to do. There were seven more fights through to 1995, when he lost to the unremarkable Fred Houpe in front of his own St. Louis fans. The descent had been utterly tragic.

His promoter at the time, Steve Frank, felt Spinks might have gone into the ring in his last two fights either drunk, high, or both. Houpe, who had been something of a warm prospect seventeen years earlier, was returning after a huge layoff. He had not fought since 1978, but Leon was washed up. The hourglass finally ran out. "His balance was gone, his reflexes were shot. I cringed anytime I saw his name on a list of fights," said boxing manager Jackie Kallen.

Leon was in such a bad way that not only was he visibly struggling but he was flunking neurological exams. He dragged one leg, was getting lost, and was losing his memory. He was told that, while it was from boxing, the alcohol wasn't helping. Dementia was closing in and he couldn't be left by himself. He wound up in a homeless shelter and lived a hard, lonely, and empty life.

Then he found work for low pay sweeping out Kiel Auditorium, a place he'd once boxed as an upcoming pro several decades earlier. He had lost it all. The money. The friends. The hangers-on.

In 2019, his voice was deep, gruff, and gravelly. His words often tended to run into each other or form one longer sound. We made small talk. I asked how long he'd been living here, how Michael was—"doing good. I still see him"—and we reverted back to Sam. Finally, Brenda yelled from another room that she wouldn't be long. Leon perched unsteadily on a stool by a breakfast bar. I sat next to him, earning Sam's approval. By this point, he and I were becoming firm friends.

Leon remained skeptical, though his welcome had been warmer than I had anticipated. He sat there shaking. It looked like he was tapping his feet and bobbing his head to music but there was none.

Brenda came in and smiled. We hugged and I thanked her for having me. She offered me a spot at the dining table, for the three of us to sit around, and Leon took off in the opposite direction. He staggered slowly away, muttering under his breath, and before I knew it the Olympic gold medalist from the 1976 Games was gone. Worse still, it was because of me. Leon had not taken kindly to my embrace of his wife and stormed off at low speed toward the bedroom in a jealous sulk. Brenda tried to reassure me and scolded herself for her own insensitivity. She and I made our way over to the dining table, with Leon nowhere to be seen despite her urging. I said it was quite fine in the hope he may reemerge while I was there, or that she may have the clout to persuade him at some point.

We walked through the open-plan living room, which had the furniture pushed back against the wall to make the floor space clearer for Leon, and talked over the loud TV. I had no idea whether I had really upset Leon, whether he didn't want any part of me because he knew I was writing a book about brain injuries and he was a subject, or if he didn't know what I was doing there and wasn't interested. I wanted to have a glimpse of what it was like to see and talk to someone with advanced-stage CTE and see what life was like for their primary caregiver.

Brenda offered me a bottle of water and we sat down and she told me how life is. "Stressful," she began.

Brenda didn't know Leon at the height of his fame, around the time of the Olympics or early in his pro career, but they had been together twenty years and had shared a modern-day love story, laced with tragedy and upset that had the archetypal highs and lows. She began to recount their time together. They met in 2000 and Leon soon moved in with her at her home in Nebraska. He earned money sweeping floors at the YMCA, working on school buses, and unloading trucks. They moved to Las Vegas in 2011 and married there.

"We met in Branson, Missouri, and I worked for the Radio City Rockettes and they had a show there," she smiled. "I worked in wardrobe, and one summer I went back just to see my friends and we went to this country-and-western bar and my friends and I were sitting in the back because it was really packed and the band stopped playing and said, 'And now Leon Spinks has entered the building.' And I said, 'Oh my God, do you know who that is?' They didn't know who it was, but I grew up in a boxing family so I knew who the boxers were and I went up and started talking to him and that's how we met."

So what did she say to capture the attention of a man whom women had thrown themselves at for years? Brenda grinned. She was clearly moved by the recollection of a simpler time. "Okay, this is crazy," she began. "I said, 'I think I met you before.' When I was fifteen I came to Las Vegas—and I couldn't remember the year at the time—I came out here to see Tony Orlando and I remember my dad saying, 'There's a big fight in Vegas, I wish I could go.' My parents never went anywhere, but my dad loved boxing and when I was leaving I remember running through the airport, trying to get to my plane, and I saw all these women screaming and this guy holding his belt and I thought, 'That must be the guy about to fight.' So I ran over there, asked to take a picture and he said, 'Yeah.'"

Fast-forward a few years. "I said [to Leon], 'Did you become the champion in the late 1970s?' And he said, 'Yeah.' I said, 'In Las Vegas?' 'Yeah.' And I said, 'Oh my God, I think I met you.' I said, 'Isn't that weird, we meet again?' So I was calling everybody and saying, 'you're never going to believe who I met.' Anyway, a couple of days later, my brother called me back and said it wasn't Leon Spinks I had met [in Vegas years earlier], it was Larry Holmes. But that's how we met and we just became friends."

Asked what her first impressions were, Brenda summed up the kind of emotions that help marriages work for decades rather than single figures. "I liked him," she said, her eyes hinting at watering. "I thought he was cute. I think he looks better now than he did then."

That's the secret. Because Leon Spinks might not be the catch now that he was then, but Brenda sees the same man and she loves him dearly. They face daily trials and struggles but they do so together.

Asked to describe how things are now she stops to consider her response carefully. "They're stressful," she again says after some contemplation. "It's just stressful because it's harder for him to get around. In 2014 he almost died. He was signing autographs and I was giving him sandwiches . . . and there must have been a bone in one of them or something. I didn't know this and he had a slither of a chicken bone that went into his intestines and he's taking coumadin [a blood thinner] so they had to do emergency surgery. That was successful; however, he started bleeding internally and then he went into a coma and that was hell. He had six surgeries in two weeks and they didn't know . . . I mean, you've just got to stay positive. Then after he was in a coma for two weeks he was in ICU [intensive care unit] for two months, then they put him on the floor for a week but they couldn't handle him on the floor, so then he had to go to a nursing home for two months. Then he went to rehab for about two and a half weeks."

Brenda was with him every step of the way, holding his hand, saying prayers, supporting his every breath—and unsure whether one of them would be his last. "I had to be there all the time," she remembered. "He had tubes in and all over him and he would pull them out. You know when they put that tube down your throat? He pulled that out probably twenty or more times. They'd call me when I'd leave. I mean, I slept in a cot in there and it was just horrible. And it was all the way on the other side of Las Vegas and we were moving at the time and thank God Rose Norton [wife of former heavyweight champion Ken] came and she and her daughter and my son moved my whole house out because I had to be at the VA."

Leon made money from his name. Where he once used it to headline big-fight cards, he then used the Spinks brand to pad an up-and-coming prospect's record as he slid into mediocrity and then obscurity. He then used it to sit and sign autographs on photos and memorabilia for fans and collectors, often in Las Vegas but sometimes further afield.

That is not without its challenges, of course. "It's a little harder," Brenda explained, still no sign of Leon, who has had to relearn the alphabet. "Because you know people want him to write all this stuff and that's more difficult. And so you need to write it down so he can do it correctly and sometimes his moods . . . you know, they rush you around when you're doing these autograph signings. We went to one in Chicago and our flight was screwed up. We were in the airport all day and we ate a little, but then you can't eat much when you're flying because the airplanes are too small to use the bathroom. It is stressful, but then he was in a bad mood when we got to the signing because he was hungry. I said, 'Can we go somewhere so we can get him something to eat?' And they wanted to rush us there and, and . . . we're slow. And they had some food back there, snacks, and once he eats he's much better. But the mood thing is sometimes hard."

Have the swings become more volatile as either he's deteriorated or as time has gone on? "I guess he's always had his moods, but it's a little more difficult now to make him understand that we've got to get this done, then we will do something else," she continued.

Yet Leon still has it within him to be charming, to please the fans, to make their day. They might leave—mourning the once-bright champion that he was—but they will have witnessed his trademark toothless grin, given him a hug, or heard him vaguely recall the night he shut up "The Greatest."

"Oh they love him," Brenda happily sighed. "The boxing fans are always excited to meet him and he likes that."

But when the crowds disperse, Brenda is left with a tired man who is an old sixty-five. His mileage in the ring (and out of it) has had a torturous effect on his health, culminating in that painstaking 2014, which Brenda conceded has irreparably slowed him down. "His walking is not as good," she lamented. "He uses a walker now a lot of the time, his balance is worse, but he's sixty-five years old, too. And we were exercising a lot more before, but we're trying to get back into shape." Her use of "we" rather than "Leon" or "he" signifies exactly how much she shoulders the burden.

Leon has been part of the Professional Fighters Brain Health Study, but some of the tests are too complex for a man who now doesn't have a mobile phone because of the routine challenges it presents and who finds cognitive exams taxing, not least because he struggles with the iPads they have to be completed on. No sooner has he got the hang of the device than the test is over. He also struggles to stay still for MRI scans.

Sometimes he is told that his reaction times for certain tests are improving and Brenda takes some solace in that. "So maybe they're getting better, I don't know," she said, with more hope than expectation. The prognosis for Leon was not good, but Brenda remained upbeat and encouraged. She was unsure that the stroke of 2014 was the lowest ebb.

"That was hell," she went on. "It scares me. Things scare me. I'm overprotective of him, I know I am. He used to be a drinker but he drinks nonalcoholic beer now [he isn't always informed of that part] and a lot of people don't know that. They think he's still drinking. But he really loves being out talking to people. Today he woke up in a different mood."

It was at that point Brenda figured there should be three of us around the table rather than two. "Come on Leon, I've got you a beer out here," she shouted.

He steadily emerged, opting to prop himself back up at the bar in a mini act of defiance. The nonalcoholic beer started to flow. We said we'd talk boxing.

"Hmm," he agreed nonchalantly.

"Who was the best you fought?"

"The best I fought? I fought Ali, for one thing."

"What set him apart, what made him special?"

"I don't know. Kicking his ass I guess."

Brenda began to help him along. "Maybe because he was supposed to be 'The Greatest,' right?"

"Yeah, well he was. But he couldn't end up doing shit."

"You didn't do a whole lot of training certainly for the rematch," I asked, referring back to his reputation of being a good-time guy. "There was a story that as Ali was waking up to go training, you saw him on your way back in from a night out, is that right?"

"Yeah. I'm trying to get his ass before he kicks my ass."

Then Leon spoke in glitches, a scratched CD on repeat. For a few minutes, even with Brenda trying to help him navigate questions, he wound up talking about Ali regardless of what he was being asked.

"He was trying to do his thing and I was too busy trying to whoop his ass."

Then: "In the first fight, Ali tried to be crazy and he tried to draw me out and kick my ass, but I wouldn't let him do it."

"Did you like him?"

"No, I didn't like the motherfucker."

Brenda laughed, knowing her man was back in fight mood. "Oh, yes you did," she protested.

"I didn't like no Ali."

"You always told me he was your idol."

"He was bullshit. Ali talked shit."

Leon did not mean it.

"Did you like Joe, Smokin' Joe?" I asked, figuring that if he was not an Ali guy today then maybe he had a soft spot for Ali's greatest rival.

"No, I didn't like Joe either."

Brenda laughed again. "He's lying."

"I ain't lying. How the hell are you going to say I'm lying when I was the motherfucker in the ring?"

"But you didn't fight Joe Frazier," his wife countered.

"No. That's what I'm saying. I didn't fuck with him."

"I have the greatest picture of me, Leon, and Joe," Brenda added. "They always had a riot together those two, when they did signings together."

"Talking shit. Talk shit," Leon cut in disapprovingly. Brenda made it lighthearted. Leon was only playing.

Knowing Spinks had sustained so much damage through his career I inquired who had hit him the hardest.

"All of the motherfuckers were hard punchers, I ran good," he went on. "That's all. I was too busy trying to get away so those motherfuckers couldn't put their hands on me and I was like, 'Ha ha, fuck you.' That's the way it was. But you'd go to the ring, these guys were trying to kill you and I was trying to save my ass."

He was back on loop, talking about his tactics of hitting and running, hitting and running. Some of it could be understood, much of it couldn't. Brenda seemed to know. It was almost as if there was a verbal shorthand Leon spoke that only she could translate, a one-way dialect she was nearly fluent in.

"Did you enjoy your boxing days?"

"Yeah, I enjoyed it a whole lot," Leon said, as if it was a stupid question. "They were trying to cut me off, and I was trying to run to the side. Motherfucker, how you going to catch me now. Boom, boom, boom, and run."

"Did you prefer the amateurs or the pros?"

"I liked the amateurs. You could kick ass and run away, but when it came to the pros it was crazy, it was different."

Then he was stuck again, on Ali, on hitting and moving, for several minutes.

"Some said you didn't fulfill your potential because you were a party guy?"

"A party guy? I don't know what kind of party I went [to]. I wasn't no party animal."

"Did you take your training camps seriously?"

"Yeah."

Then he went off about Ali again.

"I was ready."

"Did you want Cory [his son] to fight?"

"No, I never did, but he had the confidence to go in there and do it and he did. He's on that same kick. . . ."

"Do you wish you'd retired earlier?" Leon's decline was long, sad, and tragic.

"No."

Brenda knew that his final run of fights was costly, not just to his win-loss record but to the condition he found himself in later in life.

"I do," she said, intercepting the question. "I think that he fought too long. I wasn't in his life then. People loved you because you were a fun guy. . . ."

"If you could do it all again, would you do it?"

"Yeah. Yeah, because I knew how to run. That's the main thing. Hit the motherfucker four or five times, run over to the side, and when the motherfucker got closer, grab him."

I asked what he thought about Muhammad Ali's decline in health and his public battle with Parkinson's. Leon seemed almost unaware and didn't really know what to say, so Brenda stepped in. "I don't know if he really knows what condition he was in before he passed away," she told me, then she turned to Leon, adding, "He had Parkinson's disease."

"Well, I heard he had Parkinson's disease," Leon concurred. Then the former champion was talking about their fight again, running, grabbing, smack talk, and so forth.

"Do you like people coming up and getting you to sign stuff and take pictures?"

"Yeah, I like it."

"Leon, let's change the subject," Brenda went on, switching it up. "I was just thinking, tell him what your life is like. We live in Las Vegas, this is our house, and you like living here, right?"

"I like it. I enjoy it. I get along with people."

"Okay Leon, do you and I have fun when we go out and do stuff?"

"Oh yeah. But we don't fuck with nobody."

Sam the Labrador stood up and walked to Leon. He's a skilled dog. Brenda dropped her glasses accidentally. "Sam, pick them up for me."

He dutifully leaned over, collected them in his mouth, and placed them in Brenda's open hand.

Spinks had been given Sam. As a former Marine, he was entitled to a service dog because of his ailing health. Sam is an America's VetDog.

"Sam, he's our son, and he's a little bit spoiled," Brenda admitted.

"Is Leon a dog lover?"

"He changes his mind a lot, and he loves Sam, but the weird thing is they trained Sam to listen to me because sometimes Leon's hard to understand. And now Sam won't listen to me, I have to say 'Leon, tell him to do this' and he says it and Sam does [it], so he knows he's taking care of Leon. That's his main guy. He loves Leon. If Leon kisses me or something, he gets jealous, he's in here trying to jump up and kiss Leon."

"He's alright," agreed Leon.

Then Brenda changed tack again. "There's something I wanted to tell you," she said, looking at me to make sure I was concentrating, as if she had a message for people in the same situation as her. "When Leon wakes up, mornings are hard for us because he gets out of this deep sleep, he's been sleeping all night, and he's disorientated. Sometimes he feels lost a little bit, which I feel is very sad. But I find that music . . . he knows the words to every song on earth. He can start singing it when he hears it, and he loves John Denver and when he hears it, it just puts him in a better mood in the morning. I think it's because it's soothing, because he loves to dance, music is a big thing in his life. And that's one of the reasons we're together, we loved to dance. I'd go to work, I'd meet him after work, we'd go to party, we'd go to karaoke. . . ."

"We did crazy shit," Leon interjected.

"That's why we are together, because we're both sort of crazy. I was a singer, he was a dancer and he was my biggest fan. He would come and dance in front of the stage and I'd sing disco songs. I had a whole bunch of songs, but music definitely. . . . We go to see Tony Orlando, he was the best man at our wedding. And he'll be here [in Vegas], we go to all of his shows, and he says, 'Leon, I don't know how Brenda drags you to this show every night.' But I like taking him to music stuff."

Then there's the medication, prescription and otherwise. Seventeen pills a day, twelve in the morning and five in the evening, including one to help him sleep. They are carefully set out and placed into pill boxes, by Brenda, separated into times and dates.

Then there's other medicine. Marijuana is now legal in Nevada. In fact, former world heavyweight champion Mike Tyson—who once spectacularly tore through Leon's brother Michael in just ninety-one seconds in the biggest fight of 1988—has opened up his own commercial ranch.

Leon may have been on it for years but now its purpose is different. A joint can make or break a day.

"It's amazing what it turns him into," Brenda said, having carefully debated whether to mention it. She explained it's not a recreational, party element; it can just alter his outlook. "You can really have a conversation with him because I can talk to him and it's like we met twenty years ago. It calms him down. He's fun, he's happy. I was going to let him have some before you came, but I didn't know whether I should or not."

She has not always been an advocate, far from it. "I've thrown away bags of pot," she said. "I've put them in the toilet, I've done everything because I thought it was the worst thing ever, but I've totally changed my mind." She doesn't partake, but admits that Leon is used to it and has likely done it most of his life.

"Has boxing helped you?" I asked her, aware at the lack of a union, a pension fund, or any other support network that helps retired fighters around the world.

"The WBC has," Brenda replied quickly. "And they are wonderful. Mauricio [Sulaiman] is an amazing person."

"How about the sport itself, has it helped him or both of you?"

"It's his career. We've been a lot of places," she replied, scratching around for positives.

"How much do you love Brenda for what she does?"

"A whole lot. Yeah. I do," Leon admitted, his voice lifting at the end.

Frankie Pryor had talked of how Brenda and Rose Norton had helped her with Aaron, and how grateful Frankie was that Brenda and Leon travelled to Cincinnati to see "The Hawk" be laid to rest.

"We help each other out," Brenda continued. "Rose has been here a lot to help me out. It was terrible when Ken passed away because everything just changed. We'd spend weekends together, those guys would carpool together and she'd drive them to work [autograph signings] and I'd pick them up or vice versa, and those two became good friends. We'd go to their house, because Ken didn't like to go places, and Leon and Ken would sit in chairs and watch TV and we just had fun."

But a wider support system, helping with education and assistance, has not been in place for them. Worse than that, Leon has been on the receiving end of the kind of cruel teasing and taunting that boxing stereotypes have historically drawn, of fighters suffering from the effects of their careers. It's not often other sports stars are on the end of CTE gags and nastiness.

"I was so pissed," Brenda recalled of one particularly unpleasant example. "We did a radio interview in Nebraska and we had to get up really early in the morning, you know how those morning shows are, and these guys Todd and Tyler . . . I had to wake Leon out of bed and he didn't have his teeth in then and he was really hard to understand. . . . He had a manager back then who said he had to do this interview. And I never listened to this station, but they made so much fun of him saying, 'Oh, you can tell he's punch-drunk, you couldn't tell what he was saying.' And all they did was . . . they took his voice and they made commercials and they made fun of it, and it was horrible. People said I should call them, and I called them but they don't care. We've had a lot of crap like that."

The former world heavyweight champion, who ruled when the person who held that title was the most powerful man in all of sports, was being bullied and publicly humiliated because of the damage he'd sustained over the years.

On Leon's huge hands now he wears a wedding ring, a Marine Corps Boxing Hall of Fame ring, and a Nevada Boxing Hall of Fame ring.

Brenda is working on home improvements to make things easier for Leon, and she has amassed memorabilia to create his own Hall of Fame room of memories. Sometimes she has to turn down Leon's services for engagements depending on both what the demands are and whether her husband is up to it. "We never had until last year, but we had to cancel two because he's on a blood thinner. So if his blood pressure is not correct, if it's too high, I'm not going to fly, and I was so stressed out I couldn't do it. Sometimes it's very stressful taking care of people, being a caregiver. We were doing too much and I just couldn't do it. I had a lot of back pain because he's such a big guy. I was pushing him round in a wheelchair when we went out, helping him get up and down, because he has a hard time with that. My goal is to make this house handicap accessible, because I can't live in a nursing home again. That was the worst. I sold my house in Nebraska and put all the money into this house. . . ."

They are also trying to get help from grants. Boxing will do nothing. With multimillion-dollar paydays an almost monthly occurrence on the Strip a few miles north, it shuns some of its highest-profile heroes. Leon, perhaps alongside former welterweight champ Thomas Hearns, may be the most famous severe-case CTE sufferer in the sport.

There are more pictures to go up in the house but when you walk in for the first time there's a huge portrait of Leon—well beyond life-size—in his fighting days in a boxing pose, and there are framed shots of his biggest nights, winning Olympic gold and toppling Ali.

I shook Leon's hand to bid him farewell. I was careful not to hug Brenda again, and she walked me to the door. I patted Sam goodbye and he turned his attention to Leon, who lowered his head toward his boy and was licked repeatedly flush in the face by his adoring friend.

"Does he ever get frustrated?" I asked Brenda of her husband, the former world heavyweight king, as we walked toward the door.

"Sometimes he gets scared, because he doesn't know," Brenda replied, sadness and resignation in her eyes. You wouldn't ever imagine a heavyweight champion would ever be afraid. "The short-term memory is bad. But he likes watching himself, his fights. The first Ali fight and the Olympics. That's pretty much what we've got."

Before I leave, Brenda has one last thing to show me. Hung on the wall is a painting. It is bright, colorful, humorous, deep, mesmeric. It is set by the sea and on the shoreline is a stairway that leads up and out over the ocean. There are plants and shrubbery on the borders on either side of the sandstone bricks that lead up to the light among the clouds. It winds this way and that and then disappears into the sky. It leads to heaven. On the other side of the bay are a couple of trees shaped like cocktail glasses and there are three characters. Perhaps the most inconsequential is a green olive, with a harp in one arm and a halo over its head. It is near the bottom of the stairs and is likely playing for those fortunate enough to make their way up. The two central characters are two other green olives. One, with a halo and wings, is pulling another up, while the other seems to be resisting the help and instead choosing to go down into a stairway that spirals deep beneath the beach. There's a sign with arrows pointing down. "Helluva party" it says.

"I love this painting. This is me and Leon," Brenda sighed, pointing at the olives. "We both love olives and Michael Godard actually painted this for us. This is me trying to pull Leon out," she smiled, pointing at the two nearer the bottom than the top.

We both stop and stare a while at the artwork. There is silence. Brenda might be looking at "her and Leon" nearer the bottom but it's easy to stare up into the glowing clouds, and one cannot help but think that Leon is fortunate to have her on his journey to the top of the stairwell. Not everyone is lucky enough to have a Brenda. Not every fighter has such a dependable, affectionate figure to fall back on, organize their affairs, love them, cherish them, humor them, tolerate them, and support them. You see fighters like Leon on their own. Great champions, fallen warriors, helpless, laughed at, mocked, spat out, cast aside, forgotten, and helpless. Leon might have won Olympic gold and a world title. He might have headlined in Las Vegas and have become a worldwide celebrity. But these days, he has what he really needs. He has his Brenda, and for that he should be truly grateful.

* * *

Leon Spinks died about eighteen months after my visit. He had prostate cancer and was sixty-seven.

AFTERWORD
NOTHING FUCKS YOU HARDER
THAN TIME

I t comes to all, or almost all.

Moods, depression, anxiety, highs, lows, self-esteem, self-awareness, ego can all be damaged through repetitive trauma. That can change your outlook on life and, as a consequence, it can change your direction and alter your decisions.

I wonder if I am damaged. I'm forty. I can be moody. I can be emotional. I can get cranky. My temper can be short, though I've worked to contain all of that through fitness, reading, and moving out to the countryside where I find peace in daily walks with my dogs in the forest. But I was an amateur for ten years. I only had a handful of fights. I was stopped, but never knocked down—not that that matters. There are four or five guys I could tell you I boxed more than a hundred rounds with. My defense was abysmal. That is a lot of punches. I took some blows to the head that really hurt, and some of them I didn't shake for several weeks. And my memory plays tricks on me at times. I used to have a schoolboy knowledge of boxing, but now I wonder if I'm falling into the bracket of "forgotten more than I will ever know."

Maybe it's age?

There could, of course, be many reasons behind it. But I remember once, after driving back from a fight in the west of England (stopped in the second or third round in a Fight of the Night contender) that I drove clean over a roundabout and did not think anything of it. In fact, I thought I was being clever. That Saturday night, I had taken a left hand to the crown of my head when coming in underneath my taller opponent. I saw some patchy bright colors, felt my knees buckle, and the pain did not subside for a few days. It certainly was not helped when I was back in the gym sparring on Monday.

Then, one time when I was sparring with some of the pros in Kevin Rooney's Catskill Boxing Club in upstate New York, I was clobbered harder than I can ever recall being hit, even harder than any time I've stood up in a cramped space and accidently banged my head. My legs bolted firmly to the mat, like I was some kind of robot screwed in the floor, and from where I had been hit so cleanly on the jaw I remember my head tilting. I was stricken, frozen solid like a block of ice, looking at the light hanging above the ring. A volley of punches came my way. I clumsily swiped back and the round passed.

The next day, the other fighters and I did our roadwork. I had a splitting headache from the sparring. It was not the sort of migraine pain you get around your temples but toward the top and back of my head. It was like my brain was loose within my skull and, as we ran up the mountains and along the sweeping roads, it felt as though there was a rattle in my head.

The next day we sparred again and it was hard. With hindsight, I believe I was concussed. But when Rooney called me into the ring what could I say? I was trying to make a name for myself. I could not take a battering in sparring one day and opt not to box the next. I would look like a wimp. What are you going to say? "My head hurts from boxing yesterday?" Of course it hurts. It's boxing. You get hit on the head. It's the fight game. Heroic boxers have fought through infinitely worse. I said nothing and boxed, but my timing was off. I felt lethargic and flat. My head felt a great deal worse after the four rounds, too. That rattle did not completely leave through most of the summer, and I continued to train in New York, Atlantic City, and other places. And I wasn't boxing any better. I was still rubbish. I was still getting hit all the time.

I doubt any of that did me much good.

There were periods when I felt my speech slowed and was not as fluid as I would have liked, but I haven't boxed in years and don't make the same observations. That said, there have been fighters I've interviewed over the years who seemed to be slurring and on the way to a very uncertain future only to talk with more clarity in retirement—once they stopped getting hit in the head.

My father had Parkinson's before he passed away in 2012 at the age of seventy-eight. How do I feel about that, since I've taken a few thousands lumps around the head and may also have a predisposition to an illness those said lumps could trigger?

Maybe the research is not there, but the weight of numbers is sobering.

Something Chris Nowinski said to me in Boston has stayed with me. "The real tragedy of boxing and MMA is 90 percent of the damage is coming in sparring when you're not getting paid, or more," he stated. "And you could lower your exposure by over 90 percent if you change how you train. Micky Ward was the first guy who taught me that. He said he used to spar with headshots multiple days a week thinking it made him tougher for taking head blows. And we tried to tell his story when he pledged his brain that Micky, the toughest guy ever, is telling you to stop doing this. Nobody cared."

And then there's another of boxing's modern evils to contend with: performance-enhancing drugs. Fighters are stronger, hitting harder, potentially fitter, and therefore feasibly inflicting more damage than ever before on one another. It's become a huge issue and probably worthy of a book in its own right.

Often, in researching this book, I was told by a journalist, historian, and/or fighter not to forget a certain boxer who had suffered, not to leave them out. The problem was that would turn this book into a list. In arguably the definitive book about the concussion crisis in the NFL, *League of Denial*, an initial scene portrays Mike Webster—an all-time great player who had it all but lost everything—being pitied as he stumbled through his Hall of Fame induction speech.

I've been going to Canastota, home of the International Boxing Hall of Fame, since 2000. Back then, in my youth, I was blinded by the big names and thought nothing of fighters struggling to talk, walk, asking me—a penniless visitor—for handouts. I had not connected any dots. The only thing I knew was what everyone else knew: that fighters who had sacrificed so much often wound up with nothing. That's a stereotype I've been aware of since childhood, that fighters go broke. I had not wondered why or how, just accepted the notions of entourages, flashy cars, mansions, and possibly alcohol and drugs. That was it, surely. How could there be more to it than the stories we've been told since the sport began?

Well, I hold onto a different truth now, be it proved or not. In almost twenty years of visiting "boxing's hometown" and attending numerous other annual functions, I've seen the decline of fighters I looked up to, some I idolized and some I've known. And I will keep seeing it, I do not doubt. The next wave will be fighters I've watched and become friendly with. Then it will be fighters who I have covered from their debut. Then it will be fighters who weren't born when I started writing about the sport. The brutal wheel will keep turning, and fighters will keep getting spat out, broken and damaged.

They will be asked to pose, staring vacantly into cameras, to sign autographs with pens they cannot control, using letters they can scarcely remember. This is not "all," but it will be some, and more than a boxing man like me should care to admit.

You cannot blame everything on CTE. But what if it is an important factor? What if it is a difference maker? What if it is stopping lives at thirty-five years of age? Maybe not causing an overwhelming physical deterioration or debilitation but ripping away momentum, ambition, hope, and opportunity while replacing it with depression, anxiety, volatility, and emptiness.

Something needs to be done. Too often boxing momentarily is faced with a tragedy. There are sporadic pieces of how "depression is a serious issue," that we can't let another fighter die or commit suicide in vain, that "something needs to be done." Perhaps a GoFundMe page is set up and pushed by friends, family, and ex-fighters on social media before focus switches to the next money-spinning pay-per-view event, the next young prospect, the next failed drug test or political dispute, and we forget about the poor victim as the scrap heap mounts. Nothing is done. Heads were briefly turned and then it's passed. Forgotten. Footnoted. Used as a reference when the next tragedy occurs. Then the cruel cycle repeats. But if brain injuries are a major cause of the issues fighters face over time, then the sport needs to do all it can to mitigate the risks. It must educate and take its foot off the box-office-bonanza treadmill and make it safer.

Then things like what happened with English middleweight Nick Blackwell might not happen.

Blackwell, from Trowbridge in England, is a tragic case. He admitted to being hurt—probably concussed, badly—in sparring by George Groves just days before he fought Chris Eubank Jr. He was hospitalized with a brain bleed after his fight with Eubank, and while he would never fight again, he made a decent recovery. Then, months later, he sparred against his doctor's advice. This time he emerged only in part from the coma, and his life was changed forever. Blackwell had a lack of education. So did anyone who knew about the Groves sparring session and certainly those who supervised his ill-conceived spar after his initial brain bleed.

You cannot predict who will suffer, but to extend some kind of education about long-term risks to fighters and their squads should decrease the amount of stupid decisions that are too often taken.

In an interview with Sky Sports after his loss to Andy Ruiz in 2019, Anthony Joshua was asked whether the rumors that he had suffered a concussion in training were true. "I don't know what concussion is," he replied. Was it bravado? Either way, it was a missed opportunity on his part to educate about a degenerative killer and if he, the heavyweight champion of the world, didn't know what it was, it does not reflect well on his team, who are supposed to be looking out for him. All fighters should know about the risks of boxing, both chronic and acute. In 2019, to not know is simple negligence.

Fighters who fail drug tests are told to know what they are putting into their body. But boxers should also be told what is happening to their body and what might be happening to their brains. If you don't understand what concussion is, you don't understand the risks. Everything else is lip service. Second-impact syndrome, where a brain that might have recently been damaged in some way is put back in the firing line, is one of the significantly high-risk ways of sustaining an injury that your brain will never recover from. The first blow might be like an earthquake but the foundations in the brain are still standing. The second impact may only be a comparative aftershock but the foundations crumble, beyond repair. A fighter may feel okay after the first. They might never be the same again after the second.

Some fighters feel they have dodged the bullet and retired unscathed, but only time will truly tell. Who can forget the image of former world light-heavyweight champion Freddie Mills arguing the case for boxing as he'd married well, wore flashy clothes, drove fast cars, and lived in a big house only for his life to descend into chaos and end either as a murder or suicide victim?

And maybe some of the fighters who had hard bouts will be okay. Maybe.

And now I reflect on my earliest visits to the International Boxing Hall of Fame, a place that has become like a second home to me. I remember wondering why Matthew Saad Muhammad, barely fifty, was struggling to walk and talk, why the great Iran Barkley was so overweight and hitting me up for $10 for a picture, and why I was stunned at how Leon Spinks struggled to have dialogue with me.

I had not looked for a common denominator, or I did not want to see one.

It was like a scrapyard of high-price vintage cars that had decayed over time. It was heartbreaking. And the Hall of Fame treats the fighters wonderfully well. It gives them more days in the sun when otherwise they would be forgotten, but it's a fan's guilty pleasure—posing for a picture with someone who is looking emptily into a camera, habitually holding up a shaking fist in a fighter's pose or watching them sign a scarcely legible scrawl.

In the early 2000s, I visited former light-heavyweight contender James Scott in Northern State Prison, Newark, where he was serving a near thirty-year sentence for a murder he contended he never committed. He would reel off dates, historical facts, and we spoke at a brisk pace for more than an hour. When he was finally released in 2005, he began helping train youngsters in a gym in Trenton. By the time ESPN visited him to record a podcast in early 2017, he could no longer even talk. Yes, he was older and it could be attributed to any kind of disease or illness that you choose. But whatever medical issue you want to pin it on, it was another ex-boxer who, in years after retirement, became a human being who had become almost frozen in the outside world. He died in a nursing home in May 2018, aged seventy-one.

There is a line in the TV series *Game of Thrones*, "Nothing fucks you harder than time." That's true in boxing. And anyone who has read my book *The Road to Nowhere* knows I was exposed to this a long time before I knew what I was writing about. That book documented me travelling around the United States, looking for lost champions who had all but vanished. My findings were often tragic.

One who didn't seem symptomatic then was a superb middleweight from the 1960s, Joey Giambra. In retirement he had written a book, driven a cab, and he lived happily with his English bull terrier in Las Vegas. But his health eventually faltered and he became part of Dr. Bernick's fighter study.

"There were side effects that you might have seen with CTE and basically after a big stroke we were trying to get him to recover," said his son, Joey Jr. "He had a major stroke, a pulmonary embolism, and pneumonia all at the same time, and this was almost when he was in his late seventies."

The family dedicated their time and money to getting him fit and healthy. They thought the old man could win one last fight. He battled on after two more strokes for a further decade.

"We really thought he was going to get better," added daughter Gina. "He would bounce back and be how he used to be." Giambra's children now want to raise awareness about brain injuries in boxing and hope the sport ups its game, too.

The first thing that needs to be done is to change the stigma, to make sure that CTE is not looked down on, and that "punch-drunk" is no longer a dirty phrase.

"I hate those words," Joey Jr. said. "Dad hated that. You could call him any name in the book, [but if] you call him 'punchy,' he didn't like it. They thought he did suffer neurologically from boxing but he was good at hiding it."

Gina continued, "When we were younger, looking back at symptoms, he had short-term memory loss when we were children and he was in his early-to-mid and late forties, so there was forgetfulness. He was never mean, ever. He was always a happy guy. There was never a volatility side to him."

More people in the sport need to get conformable talking about the uncomfortable and having the hard conversations, but there are signs that it is changing. For instance, social media is playing a role. Old fighters who befriend one another on Facebook and other platforms have openly talked about it. In August 2019, Rudy Cisneros, a welterweight with twelve wins and four losses, posted, "Leaving the Drs office w/Great News. . . . Boxing has done damage but not as worst as some other fighters received."

Aaron Torres, now forty-one and ten years retired from a career that saw him win sixteen and lose seven, commented on his status. "Good to hear. I on the other hand am in pain most of the day."

Rudy, now thirty-nine, replied, "Famz get checked cuz u don't want it to be late . . . bro the headaches n migraines are unbearable sometimes."

Torres replied: "I have been checked out several times. By all kinds of doctors. They can't find anything wrong. SMH."

Rudy: "It's like a ghost symptom."

Ohio's Courtney Patterson, retired after going 1-4 in the pros, joined in. "They experimented giving me different stuff to see if it work. I was like hell no. My equilibrium was off. i slurred heavy short-term memory problems. But they kept saying nothing was wrong. For years. But ok it is what it is."

Torres: "its not cool. They gave me some medicine that made me almost pass out at work."

Patterson: "man they gave me medicine that would stop me cold! I went to the hospital 1 night they gave me something they told me I would freak out in a few minutes too. I got it went home and thought ppl were trying to kill me. No you're right it ain't cool. I went to a mental place for help the dumb asses diagnosed me as depressed. What? My speech slurred I can't remember stuff from yesterday how is that the only diagnosis?! Neurologist told they couldn't find anything wrong. I was like ok yeah. I just got tired of being frustrated and being told nothing was wrong. Aaron."

They went back and forth a little then Patterson continued: "My last fight was dec '08. I been got injured in the gym but took fights and sparred anyway. I couldn't get out the way of punches. Wack ass ppl beat me. Feather fisted chumps. It was terrible"

Torres later replied: "I'm tired of the pain and feeling like shit every day. Guess that's the price we pay . . . I'm tired of it. It depresses the shit out of me. I was fine up until 2 years ago. Then everything started crashing. I've seen every type of doctor. Two E.R visits last year. I thought it was all over."

Patterson: "Im concerned about when im an old man. I know ppl way worse. I've heard the stories of meldrick Taylor. You're from philly I know you've seen up close. It is like I've done this for nothing man. I love boxing though. My last coaching was 2017 I've been working too much to be involved . . . I hate the little boys being rock em sock em robots and those lame ass coaches cheering it on. Most never put a glove on. I hate that in boxing you don't need any experience just by a license and you're a coach . . . depression shouldn't have been the only diagnosis is what pissed me off. Hell yeah it depressed me. When you show the world it doesn't."

Torres: "I've shared the ring with Mel. Great guy. Very sad what happened to him."

There is an increasing trend. Fighters are realizing. Perhaps they are learning too late, but the cycle is coming round faster, generally.

Israel Pito Cardona, retired at 36-10 and now aged forty-five, posted this in March 2016: "I enjoyed being on top of the boxing world I'm honored to be inducted to the ct [Connecticut] boxing hall of fame if I had the luck to become a multimillionaire I still wld change it in a second to not be suffering the way I am now I have CTE I can't work or drive anymore there's nothing I can do or any doctor can do to fix it I'm alone dealing with this my family my mom I'm sorry that I have to depend on u my brothers n sister I'm hoping something good comes out of all this crap to my fellow boxers or mma fighters be very carefull the only reason I'm in this fuck up situation it's cause of this fucked up sport called boxing I still love the sport but make sure U On top of ur game it's a dangerous sport."

It takes a different kind of bravery to have these discussions, to share experiences and knowledge and for fighters to be there for one another in this loneliest of endeavors, but they are vital discussions to be had.

And some of the fans are starting to notice a deterioration over time. While in Canastota in 2018 with one regular observer, he leaned over and whispered, asking whether I'd seen a former heavyweight great.

"No," I replied.

"Oh man," came the reply. "He's got it."

"Got what?" I asked.

"The death shuffle."

The fighter was around sixty years of age and maybe to the untrained eye he was not too bad. But to boxing fans who had seen him over the years, the changes were stark. The eyes were a little more sunken, the arms "swung" more rigidly, and the walking was like a slow-motion hopscotch.

And still, on the ground, at ringside and with governing bodies, you see the errors that lead to problems. Fighters not serving adequate times for suspensions, fights being stopped too late, poor treatment post-fight. . . .

In one of the top jobs in boxing journalism, I witnessed things that made me wonder if being ringside to watch was morally correct. In Herning, Denmark, I saw Carl Froch and Mikkel Kessler swapping punches—to the head—that sounded like thin gloves crashing into a side of a slab of meat. I watched Manny Pacquiao get obliterated by a Juan Manuel Marquez right hand that I thought for some moments had either devastatingly injured the Filipino icon or, worse, killed him. I was there when Amir Khan was floored and severely dazed by Breidis Prescott, and briefly, stupidly, allowed to continue before having his senses removed for a much longer period of time.

Then there was one shocking night in Las Vegas, the eve of a big fight across the Strip, when I watched a little man from the Philippines, Z. Gorres, dominate an opponent but then take a sickening shot, a straight left from a southpaw, with moments left in the fight. As he fell, his head whiplashed off the bottom rope. I was watching from a balcony and could see the whites of Gorres's eyes. They seemed to be rolling. His feet were unsteady. He was way in front on points but I felt the fight should have been stopped. He was in no position to continue and he needed to be looked after. He was allowed to see out the fight. It was like seeing a shell of a man, a very small man, with nothing left in him.

He held on for the remaining twenty seconds or so and won, but he went to his corner at the end and he could not even celebrate. His brain was swelling fast. He was losing consciousness. No one seemed to realize but me. I panicked as I wrote. I could not understand how no one else could detect what was happening. Even the referee called the fighters to the center of the ring and raised Gorres's arm. At best, Gorres was in a fog. At worst, he was ready for a far tougher fight than his Colombian opponent had given him. As he bent over to leave the ring, clearly in massive difficulty though apparently unseen by anyone else in the House of Blues but me, he continued his slow descent to the canvas. He kept falling. Everything went to black. I was tearing my hair out. He'd been in the ring, lost and abandoned, for several minutes.

He was stretchered from ringside and though he eventually woke up, he never boxed again. His dreams were over, but at least he had survived. He came through an emergency brain operation at the University Medical Center in Vegas within an hour of collapsing. Two months went by and there was further surgery to reattach the bone in the skull that doctors had removed so they could drain the blood clot from his brain. He had been away from home four months before he was able to return to his four children. He underwent a further two operations back in Cebu.

But, of course, it's not just about fight night. It's what happens down the line. I think of the fighters who have given me so many thrills and spills, some I consider friends. I wonder how they may be at events we go to over the years. Will they be the same? Will they be shaking or slurring? Will they remember their fights? Will they remember me? It's a serious subject but for too long in boxing it's been taboo.

On the way to the British Boxing Board of Control offices to interview general secretary Robert Smith and medical officer Dr. Neil Scott for this book, I was in a cab and the driver asked what my business was in Cardiff. I told him about the subject and he recommended a fighter I should speak to, a local man who'd boxed against well-known trainer Mark Tibbs. "He wasn't much good but he had a few fights," the driver, clenching his back teeth as though the subject was an awkward one to address, said. "You should see if you can talk to him, though you won't get much out of him. He's in a terrible way."

The old fighter he was talking about was fifty-six years old.

Yet punch-drunk syndrome, almost one hundred years after its first diagnosis, is seen as some kind of humiliation. It means you can't be any good. It means you're messed up. It means you walk and talk in an odd way.

You don't hear the same negative connotations about CTE in the NFL. And the very terminology around "punchy" fighters is used, in the modern-day lexicon, to insult and criticize.

On the front of newspapers worldwide in 2018, U.S. President Donald Trump, firing back at criticism from actor Robert DeNiro, pointed to the Hollywood star's portrayal of Jake LaMotta in *Raging Bull* and wrote on his social media, "Robert De Niro, a very Low IQ individual, has received too many shots to the head by real boxers in movies. I watched him last night and truly believe he may be punch-drunk." Later, he added, "Wake Up Punchy!"

As long as the term "punch-drunk" is casually used in a derisive manner, it's going to be hard to address. It will remain an elephant in the room. And as long as that's the case, it won't be treated properly because fighters and athletes won't want to admit having it. They won't want to be the person someone tuts at and says, "He's gone."

Boxing has saved more souls than it's taken. It remains a way out of poverty and trauma for thousands of men and women around the world. It builds a discipline that is hard to understand unless you've experienced it, and instills self-esteem, motivation, structure, routine, and confidence. It's transformed the lives of people headed down the wrong path and it's given hope to those who might have had none. It's turned career criminals into wise coaches who help others. It's given to many people lives they would not have had; in the words of Muhammad Ali, Aaron Pryor, and others, if they could do it all over again, even at risk of being damaged, then they would. It was their choice to make.

This book is not about the abolition of boxing but about how the culture can change to help fighters and help the sport progress. The NFL begrudgingly acted when presented with scientific information that boxing has the same access to; it's the responsibility of those in the sport to acknowledge, change, and adapt.

It's time to be open about it and time to talk about it. It's time boxing confronts its own worst problem, stops ignoring it, and steps up to address it at all levels. This is a sport of courage and it will take bravery but it's happened in football, soccer, and rugby although it should not be up to other sports to take on boxing's biggest fight.

REFERENCES

CHAPTER 1: PUNCH-DRUNK

Dr. Harrison Martland started this ball rolling in 1928. His groundbreaking medical paper, "Punch Drunk," saw the terminology accepted and he was the first man on record to discuss symptoms and patterns in fighters.

The paper, which was first produced in the October 13, 1928, issue of the *Journal of the American Medical Association* (initially published in 1883), remains poignant, which is in part why I decided to reproduce sections of it. It was a pivotal moment.

Background material for Martland was found in a January 2018 issue of *Brain: A Journal of Neurology* and in a March 1981 (Volume 2, Issue 1) copy of *The American Journal of Forensic Medicine and Pathology*. Information was also gleaned from *The Concussion Crisis: Anatomy of a Silent Epidemic* by Linda Carroll and David Rosner.

Full details of the lawsuit between Bob Fitzsimmons and the New York State Athletic Commission can be found at leagle.com (Fitzsimmons v. N. Y. S Athletic Comm.), and BoxRec was hugely helpful as always, helping to identify the fighters Martland left clues over, including Nathan Ehrlich.

Family members had left a tribute to "Uncle Nate" at www.geni.com that included details of the benefit night.

Much of the research on Ad Wolgast came from a four-part 1954 series in *The Ring* by then-editor Nat Fleischer, while interviews with boxing historian Bob Mee and bare-knuckle boxing historian Scott Burt provided plenty of color and detail.

There's much fascinating work about Joe Grim available, including a long feature from onmilwaukee.com and a June 21, 1971, *Sports Illustrated* article on "The Ironclad Punching Bag."

Gene Tunney's famous quote was cited by Martland himself, but originally came from an interview in the August 3, 1928, edition of the *New York Daily News*.

Details of Leo Lomski's curious life after boxing came from his *New York Times* obituary from November 14, 1975, and a biography on cyberboxingzone.com.

CHAPTER 2: DEMENTIA PUGILISTICA

Huge thanks to boxing writer Terry Dooley, a librarian by trade, for helping me source many crucial papers, which included the vital July 1937 J. A. Millspaugh work "Dementia Pugilistica" in the *United States Naval Medical Bulletin*.

The case of Del Fontaine is intriguing. There's a story about it in the *Milwaukee Journal* from July 19, 1935, and also more coverage about it in Ernst Jokl's book, *The Medical Aspect of Boxing*. But because Del Fontaine's real name was Raymond Henry Bousquet it seemed Jokl was trying to protect his identity and he quoted from the *Evening Standard* (September 16, 1935), "Before the court was RHB, aged 30, a Canadian boxer who fought under the name DF. He was accused of the murder of Miss HM. . . ."

He covered the Fontaine case in his "Legal Aspects" chapter.

The Osnato and Giliberti paper on "Postconcussion Neurosis—Traumatic Encephalitis" appeared in *Neurology and Psychiatry* in August of 1927, and Harry L. Parker's important work "Traumatic Encephalopathy" ("Punch Drunk") of professional pugilists, was published in July 1934 in the *Journal of Neurology and Psychopathology*.

The stories on Frank Carbone and Jimmy Flood came from the huge work by Friedrich Unterharnscheidt and Julia Taylor-Unterharnscheidt, *Boxing: Medical Aspects, while* Neil Carter's *Medicine, Sport and the Body: A Historical Perspective*, provided the information of the 1933 proposals for the NABA to introduce helmets along with Ted Broadribb suing *The Sunday Dispatch*.

Jokl's background came from several sources, including *The Medical Aspect of Boxing* and his obituary in the *New York Times* on December 21, 1997.

Jokl's book was hard to obtain but was a treasure trove of research.

It included the story of Max Baer preparing for Carnera's left hook and information on the North American Boxing Association planning to build a care home for fighters.

There was plenty on the Gans–Nelson and Nelson–Wolgast fights in the Unterharnscheidt book with additional information from *Joe Gans: A Biography of the First African American World Boxing Champion* by Colleen Aycock and Mark Scott and in *Battling Nelson, the Durable Dane: World Lightweight Champion, 1882–1954* by Mark Allen Baker.

Bowman and Blau's "Psychotic States Following Head and Brain Injury in Adults and Children" included a detailed section on traumatic encephalopathy of pugilists or punch drunk.

Background information on Bowman came from a biographical sketch in *The American Journal of Psychiatry*, April 1, 2006, while information on Blau came from his *New York Times* obituary on May 16, 1979.

The research on Ray Robinson came from his book with Dave Anderson, *Sugar Ray*, and from the HBO documentary, *The Bright Lights and Dark Shadows of a Champion*.

Again, BoxRec provided many of the stats and facts, while the final quote from Gussie Armstrong was from the November 21, 1988, issue of *People* magazine. There was more information in the *Los Angeles Times*, August 14, 1988, in the piece "Fight of His Life: Boxing Immortal Henry Armstrong, at 75, Is Enduring Tough Times Again."

CHAPTER 3: A SLICK MEDICAL CLICHÉ

Information on the Cocoa Kid, or Herbert Lewis Hardwick, came from Springs Toledo, whether it was from interviewing Toledo or taken from his brilliant book, *Murderers' Row: In Search of Boxing's Greatest Outcasts*. Again, BoxRec was the home for many of the statistics.

Information on MacDonald Critchley was obtained from The Neuro Times: A blog about neurology and neuroscience, that featured him on September 8, 2009, as well as from his obituary in the January 1998 edition of the *Journal of the American Medical Association*. His paper, "Medical Aspects of Boxing: Particularly from a Neurological Standpoint," was another key brick in this wall and was published on February 16, 1957, in the *British Medical Journal*.

G. La Cava's 1963 paper was titled, "Boxer's Encephalopathy" and was published in the *Journal of Sports Medicine and Physical Fitness*.

C. B. Courville's work was called "Punch Drunk" and appeared in the *Bulletin of the Los Angeles Neurological Society* on December 1, 1962, and on October 19, 1963, Mawdsley and Ferguson filed "Neurological Disease in Boxers" in *The Lancet*.

The October 1953 issue of *The Ring* ran a story with the headline, "Demand for Boxers Insurance Grows," while background information on Maxie Rosenbloom came from Carroll and Rosner's *The Concussion Crisis*, as well as a *Los Angeles Times* column from May 17, 1998, by Cecilia Rasmussen. There was also a graphic account of his final years in *Sports Illustrated* (April 11, 1983), entitled "How Punchy Was Slapsie Maxie?" by Jeff Wheelwright.

Information on Ralph Dupas came from the documentary, *Fighting Men of New Orleans*, and a further documentary, *The Has Beens*, narrated by Denzil Batchelor, was recorded for the BBC in 1965.

Details on Jimmy Wilde's final years came from his book, *Fighting Was My Business* which author Peter McInness added to after Wilde's passing.

Peter Heller's book, *In This Corner . . . !: Forty-two World Champions Tell Their Stories*, remains one of the great boxing books written capturing increasingly long-forgotten stars but also featuring fighters we will always remember.

Mike Silver provided some quality insight and anecdotes to accompany this chapter and Carlos Acevedo mailed me his brilliant piece on Don Jordan, "The Catastrophist: The Troubled World of Don Jordan," which was published by SB Nation on October 27, 2010.

Promoter Jack Solomons's argument for boxing was covered in the book of his rival, Dr. Edith Summerskill, *The Ignoble Art*, which referenced their ongoing debate. Freddie Mills, also referred to in that book and then at the height of his wealth and fame, was later thought to have CTE by MP Chris Evans, who was being interviewed for a story in the August 7, 2018, edition of Freddie's hometown newspaper, the *Bournemouth Echo*.

The stats of deaths in sport at the time came from Dr. Thomas Gonzalez's 1951 paper "Fatal Injuries in Competitive Sports," published on August 18 in the *Journal of the American Medical Association*.

Dr. Ira McCown, of the "slick medical cliché," wrote that controversial "Boxing Injuries" piece, which appeared in the *American Journal of Surgery* in 1959, while the demise of Johnny Bratton, Jimmy Flood, and

Johnny Saxton were covered in the Unterharnscheidt's book, *Boxing: Medical Aspects*.

Felice Leeds's excellent documentary *The Brain of a Boxer: The Story of Paul Pender*, answered plenty of questions, as did the section on Pender in the book, *The Concussion Crisis: Anatomy of a Silent Epidemic* by Linda Carroll and David Rosner.

Jokl's *The Medical Aspect of Boxing* also was used when talking about the use of the left side to corroborate a Mike Silver theory.

The background of the man many credit with the terminology, CTE, Henry Miller, came from multiple sources, including his November 9, 1965, paper "Mental Sequelæ of Head Injury," published in the *Proceedings of the Royal Society of Medicine* and a year later he wrote "Mental After-effects of Head Injury" posted in the same publication.

CHAPTER 4: THE COLLECTOR

A. H. Roberts's tome was initially an in-depth medical article ("Medical Notes in Parliament" published in the *British Medical Journal* and *Medical News* in 1962) that became a book, *Brain Damage in Boxers: A Study of the Prevalence of Traumatic Encephalopathy Among Ex-Professional Boxers*, because of how comprehensive it was.

"The Aftermath of Boxing," which presented J. A. N. Corsellis's research, was a seminal paper that created a whole new understanding about what was happening to the brain through boxing.

Information from the closure of the Corsellis Collection came from a Matthew R. Williams piece on oruen.com.

I spoke with my predecessor as editor of *Boxing News*, Claude Abrams, at several points during the process of writing this book, and some of his thoughts appear in this chapter. The Muscular Dystrophy advertisement that starred a broken Ezzard Charles can be found on YouTube and more details on Charles, his career, and his decline, came from William Dettloff's impeccable book on "The Cincinnati Cobra," titled *Ezzard Charles: A Boxing Life*. Researchers at Boston University and their work on ALS due to head trauma, "Head Trauma Linked to ALS-Like Disease," was published in *BU Today*.

CHAPTER 5: POSTER BOYS

The backbone of this chapter came from interviews with Thomas Hauser and Bobby Quarry. I was put in touch with Quarry by the prolific boxing writer James Slater. Hauser's terrific book *Muhammad Ali: His Life and Times* is illuminating about Ali's ailing health toward the end of his career and in retirement. Through Ali, he obtained records and interviews that would have otherwise remained confidential—and thus unknown.

The *Sports Illustrated* piece, "Too Many Punches, Too Little Concern," was written by Robert Hoyle and Wilmer Ames and appeared in the April 11, 1983, issue. That article was quoted several times in the chapter, while Ferdie Pacheco's lines came through Hauser and the BBC documentary *Ali: One Punch Too Many*.

Punch statistics from Ali's career came from the brilliant CompuBox book *Muhammad Ali: By the Numbers* by Bob Canobbio and Lee Groves.

Mike Silver was adamant that Ali could have done more for the CTE cause and the Quarry book referred to in this chapter is *Hard Luck: The Triumph and Tragedy of "Irish" Jerry Quarry* by Steve Springer.

The information on Ali's speech came from the October 4, 2017, paper, "Using Muhammad's Ali's Speech for Science," from the University of Melbourne, and Visar Berisha and Julie Liss who retrospectively measured the speed at which the Louisville Lip spoke at.

Again, BoxRec provided stats and an abundance of facts, and the sad Quarry–Cranmer fight can be found on YouTube.

There was a fascinating Quarry piece by Steve Wilstein (Associated Press) in the October 29, 1995, edition of the *Los Angeles Times*.

The quotes from Jim Quarry came from an interview with Kent Appell of the website Boxing247.com in 2001. The Jerry Quarry Foundation website remained a ghost town of empty promises and pledges to transform and reform a stagnant sport until it vanished from the internet during the writing of this book.

CHAPTER 6: RUSTING GOLD

I'm grateful to Earnie Shavers, Chuck Wepner, and George Foreman for their words as three of the remaining elder statesmen from that 1970s heavyweight period.

The sad tale of George Chuvalo was documented in the Canadian national press, particularly *The Star* ("The Fight Over Boxing Legend George Chuvalo") on November 3, 2017, and the *Toronto Sun* ("Boxing Legend George Chuvalo Wins First Round in Ugly Family Battle"), June 15, 2019. I interviewed Chuvalo, then in great health, in 2004. The Norton

Deadspin article ran on February 3, 2012, and I interviewed veteran New York boxing writer Jack Hirsch via email for details on Floyd Patterson, with further details from his hearing with the New York's Athletic Commission that appeared in the *New York Post* in 1998. Ernie Terrell's sister, Lovie Mickens, told the *New York Daily News*, in Ernie's obituary, that his cause of death was dementia. Information about Scott LeDoux was found in the *MinnPost*, May 5, 2010, and on TwinCities.com, May 10, 2010. Duane Bobick's wife, Deb, was quoted by the *Morrison County Record* on February 12, 2012.

CHAPTER 7: CONCUSSION
I'm grateful to Ann McKee, Chris Nowinski, and Robert Cantu for their generosity, time, and understanding. Reading the incredible *League of Denial: The NFL, Concussions, and the Battle for Truth*, by Mark Fainaru-Wada and Steve Fainaru, in many ways led me to write this book and it certainly led me to Nowinski's fascinating book, *Head Games: Football's Concussion Crisis from the NFL to Youth Leagues*. Cantu's own book, *Boxing and Medicine*, was also illuminating, and came to me courtesy of boxing writer Glynn Evans.

CHAPTER 8: THE STUDY
I was given a tour of the Lou Ruvo Clinic in Las Vegas by Christine Moorhead on June 12, 2018, and interviewed Dr. Charles Bernick via Skype on June 21, 2018, and later on the phone.

CHAPTER 9: CONTRADICTION
I interviewed Dr. Nitin Sethi at the Weill Cornell Medicine in Manhattan, New York, on June 5, 2018, and we have remained in touch. He referred to the piece, "Concussion Is Confusing Us All" in the *British Medical Journal*, Volume 15, Issue 3. I also have an application form for Sethi's study, "Quantifying Traumatically-Induced Neuroinflammation."

CHAPTER 10: CHAOS
Margaret Goodman was good enough to meet me in Las Vegas on June 11, 2018, and she also guided me to two fascinating books, her own novel, *Death in Vegas*, which gives an in-depth look at the machinations that make boxing and people in the sport tick, and a book she helped

produce while she was on the Nevada State Athletic Commission, *Ringside and Training Principles*, which is one every trainer, manager, and fighter should own but probably does not.

CHAPTER 11: DILEMMA
I've known Freddie Roach since 2008 and we have often spoken of his health and previously about the health of his relatives but we spoke extensively over the phone on June 17, 2018, for this book.

CHAPTER 12: BURIED ALIVE
I spoke with Tom Moyer on August 19, 2018. I was moved to call him having watched the 2009 documentary, *After the Last Round*, directed by Ryan Pettey, about CTE in boxing.

CHAPTER 13: LABELED
I'd known Aaron Pryor for many years in the lead-up to his passing, as well as his wife Frankie. I visited them at home in Cincinnati in 2004 and saw them regularly at the International Boxing Hall of Fame in Canastota up until Aaron's death in 2016. I interviewed Frankie for the book on August 28, 2018. I had not intended it to be for *Damage*, it was really to catch up and to see how she was doing, but when I let her know what I was writing about the topic changed direction and I learned about the wives of CTE in boxing, Frankie, Brenda Spinks, and Rose Norton.

CHAPTER 14: A WARRIOR'S BRAIN
I've interviewed Micky Ward many times over the last twenty years, including several visits to his home in Lowell when he was still an active fighter. The interview here took place in Graziano's restaurant in Canastota, New York, on June 8, 2018.

CHAPTER 15: TRAPPED
I'm hugely grateful to Ian Probert for visiting Herol Graham with me. We saw the former multiple-world-title challenger in the psychiatric unit of a London hospital on a sunny afternoon on July 4, 2018.

CHAPTER 16: RISK TAKERS
Thanks to Amir Khan, Lennox Lewis, Matt Macklin, Scott Welch, Steve Bunce, Carl Froch, Larry Merchant, Glenn McCrory, Kelly Pavlik, Christy

Martin, Gerry Cooney, Marco Antonio Barrera, Bert Cooper, John H. Stracey, George Groves, Mark Hobson, Paulie Malignaggi, Anthony Fowler, Tony Jeffries and all of the fighters who helped contribute to this chapter.

CHAPTER 17: SAFETY NETS

I visited Robert Smith at the British Boxing Board of Control offices, where we met with Neil Scott, the Board's leading medical officer. I caught up with Mauricio Sulaiman at the WBC's Convention in Ukraine in 2019, where I also interviewed Gerry Cooney. Thanks to Matt Farrago for discussing his own experiences and the work of Ring 10 and to Dave Harris for discussing his plans for a rest home for boxers.

CHAPTER 18: TEQUILA FOR BREAKFAST

Interviews with Scott Welch, Evander Holyfield, Peter Flanagan (courtesy of daughter Tina), Joe Calzaghe, Frank Bruno, and Dominic Ingle were all so very helpful. The Andre Ward quotes came from his interesting podcast with Joe Rogan.

EPILOGUE

Brenda and Leon Spinks were kind enough to welcome me into their Henderson, Nevada, home in April 2019. Frankie Pryor helped put me in contact with Brenda and I spent the good portion of that spring morning with one of boxing's best-known couples and one of boxing's best-known chronically-brain-injured fighters. Further information on Leon came from the superb book on the Spinks brothers, *One Punch from the Promised Land: Leon Spinks, Michael Spinks, and the Myth of the Heavyweight Title*, by John Florio and Ouisie Shapiro.

NOTES

[1] And this was in an era when some fighters bathed their faces in brine, a salt-and-vinegar mix, hardening their heads and toughening their skin so it wouldn't be so easy to be cut by an opponent's punches.

[2] It's difficult to be exact with fighting records from those days. Sometimes contests were exhibitions, sometimes they did not happen but records show they did, and sometimes the results did not reflect what had actually happened. That still happens today, of course.

[3] Their father had been a Golden Gloves champion in 1937 and had ten professional fights in the 1930s, winning three and boxing fifty professional rounds in all.

ACKNOWLEDGMENTS

This book has been several years in the making. Initially I wanted to write about life after boxing. It's easy to see a trend of fighters struggling in retirement but it was only after reading *League of Denial*, about the NFL's concussion crisis, that I looked deeper into boxing's own predicament.

I'd written about murder, suicides, depression, and brain injuries for years in connection with boxing. I'd said how tragic the sport was, then went back to work on the next big-fight preview. I said how something needed to change, then wrote about the next flunked drug test.

I became aware that these issues weren't going away and wanted to make it something that I, at least, didn't shrug my shoulders at and no longer winced at. Rather, I take ownership of CTE in boxing even if others don't. If I didn't, I'd be part of a problem.

Several people have helped me enormously on this journey. Lee Blasdale and Derek Andrews have been tremendously supportive. The talented Ian Probert has assisted me with some of the more challenging parts of the final manuscript and also set up our visit with Herol Graham. My friend George Zeleny also waved his red pen at some of my work and supplied some of the documentaries that were so useful in research, especially *After the Last Round*. That took me to Tom Moyer, who along with Dr. Robert Cantu, Mike Silver, and Bobby Quarry said the same thing that stuck with me while in the trenches of working on the book: "This is a great thing that you're doing," which proved to be wonderfully encouraging.

I feel extremely fortunate that I can reach out to writing giants like Thomas Hauser, Nigel Collins, and Donald McRae for support and help. I appreciate them more than they know.

Matt Christie, *Boxing News* editor, is an invaluable sounding board, as is Claude Abrams, former *Boxing News* editor. Fight manager Mike Altamura also helped me with some critical support and pointed me in the direction of some great sources.

A lot of fighters talked about something that is not comfortable to talk about, but that's important. It's vital to make the uncomfortable comfortable, to pick the scab so the sport can heal.

Some fighters have spoken to me about their concerns, some are anxious about their futures. Some have moved into media and worry about their memories on live TV, and whether their broadcasting future will be affected by their voice because they think they are starting to slur. One trainer of world champions, in deep conversation about this subject, told me to stop talking because one more piece of information would see him leave the sport and he still has a stable of top active fighters.

Of course, when you take on a project like this you need help and understanding. Kyle Sarofeen and Andy Komack at Hamilcar are a dream to work with. Not only that, but they were instantly as passionate about this subject as I was and behind the concept from the get-go. Thanks to Shannon LeMay-Finn for her patience and Carlos Acevedo and Michael Ezra for their input.

The beautiful Johanna Hancock has kept my spirits up while I've trekked around the United Kingdom, the United States, and mainland Europe trying to gather the material on these pages. Her support is priceless, and I'm consistently motivated to write well to make my children, Ben and Lois, proud of their father.

My mother, Wanda, and brother, Justin, have always been and always are supportive.

The way things worked out with *Damage*, my final destination was the brain bank in Boston.

By the time I got there, the neurologists were heroes to me as much as the fighters. Chris Nowinski shuffled his schedule to accommodate me, Dr. Robert Cantu was wonderfully helpful and fantastically interesting, and Dr. Ann McKee is a modern legend. Her assistants showed me around the brain bank and the labs. After writing about brains and CTE for so long, I was permitted to feel a brain—while dressed in medical coveralls—and then went into the laboratory to see some slides. I was shown one through a microscope. There were pink-white blotches on a red background. It was CTE. It was a defining moment for me. I became emotional. A three-year journey culminated in my coming face-to-face with the illness that has destroyed some of the greatest fighters of all time.

And I suppose, on that note, this is why I do what I do, and it's why I've done this—for the fighters. For those who have struggled, for those who are still fighting and for those who have their futures ahead of them and can now make more informed decisions about boxing, training, sparring, and retirement.

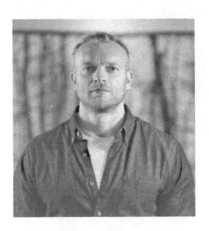

TRIS DIXON has written about boxing at all levels for more than two decades. He is the former editor of *Boxing News* and has covered the sport in more than a dozen countries across four continents. Dixon has written for *The Ring* and Boxing Scene and has worked as a boxing broadcaster for Sky Sports, BT Sport, and CNN. He authored *The Road to Nowhere: A Journey Through Boxing's Wastelands*, and ghostwrote *War and Peace: My Story* with British boxing icon Ricky Hatton. He's also the host of the popular *Boxing Life Stories* podcast, an elector for the International Boxing Hall of Fame, a member of *The Ring* ratings panel, the Boxing Writers' Club, and the Boxing Writers Association of America.

Damage is set in 10-point Sabon, which was designed by the German-born typographer and designer Jan Tschichold (1902–1974) in the period 1964–1967. It was released jointly by the Linotype, Monotype, and Stempel type foundries in 1967. Copyeditor for this project was Shannon LeMay-Finn. The book was designed by Brad Norr Design, Minneapolis, Minnesota, and typeset by New Best-set Typesetters Ltd.